Joyful
Birth

Also available
Bearing Witness: Childbirth Stories Told by Doulas

Joyful Birth

More Childbirth Stories Told by Doulas

Dr Lisa Doran, BSc, ND
& Lisa Caron, CD & PCD (DONA)

FOX
WOMEN'S
BOOKS

Dedication

This book is dedicated to my children, Jacob, Alden and Elijah.
For the joy you bring to my life every day –Lisa Doran

I dedicate this book with love and gratitude
to the memory of my mother, Mary Ann. –Lisa Caron

Cataloguing in publication data is available.
ISBN 978-1-894997-19-5
Designed and typeset by Sari Naworynski
and Susan Hannah.
Cover: Art Direction by Nuala Byles.
Printed and bound in Canada.
Published by Fox Women's Books,
an imprint of Quarry Press Inc., PO Box 1061, Kingston, Ontario
K7M 2L5 Canada www.quarrypress.com

The opinions of the contributing authors do not necessarily
reflect the opinions of the editors.

Names and stories have been changed for privacy. If they were
not changed the families gladly gave permission to tell their
stories. Some stories were told by the laboring woman herself.

Contents

Foreword

I THANK LISA CARON AND LISA DORAN for their invitation to contribute a foreword to *Joyful Birth* and for the opportunity to share, as a midwife and midwife educator, some of my reflections about their book and about birth. First, I congratulate them for inspiring women, doulas, and childbirth educators to come forward and unabashedly recount their stories of joyful birth. They have encouraged the reframing of birth as an occasion of empowerment and delight. In this book are delicious dishes, the ingredients of good cooking, menus of experiences, recipes for satisfying births, and memories that can be savored for a lifetime. *Joyful Birth* adds to a growing body of media and literature that reflects the positive rather than alienating depictions of birth that are unfortunately all-too-popular.

Within *Joyful Birth* are women's powerful stories about what was important to them during childbirth. *Joyful Birth* particularly celebrates the doula's work, her journey, learning, and impressions. It brings us testimonies by women expressing great appreciation for the continuous support and attendance of a caring doula and stories by doulas honoring women's strengths and power. The stories are simple, fresh, alive, raw, and full of colorful, sensual, and seasonal detail. They are intensely personal, recounted from feeling – and they evoke strong responses. Above all, they pay homage to women, birth, and family.

Among the many aspects of birthing that Caron and Doran illustrate as contributing to a satisfying experience is a woman's choice of birth place. I am reminded of a seminal article by Niles Newton, "The Trebly Sensuous Woman" (*Psychology Today*, 1971), which highlighted the significant role the hormone oxytocin plays in lovemaking, birthing, and breastfeeding. Newton's research showed that the release of oxytocin triggers three contracting functions: sexual excitement and orgasm, strong effective labor contractions, and stimulation of the flow of breast milk. (This simple concept was made more explicit recently in the film *Orgasmic Birth* – adapted as *Organic Birth*.) The French word for orgasm, *la jouissance*, also means 'pleasure' and 'joy'. Yes, joyful birth, when the oxytocin works well – when its effective release brings the baby and the concomitant intense feelings of well-being, satisfaction, and affection!

What is even more intriguing about this triple oxytoxic effect is that the functioning of this hormone can be inhibited by disturbance. How can one make love, labor, or breastfeed while feeling threatened or unsafe? This concept showed as well that birth happens mostly on its own, as a normal physiological function. It seems important to support a woman's right, not just to a normal physiological birth, but to an "undisturbed birth," free from anxiety, fear, and physical threat. All those associated with a birth do well to support and facilitate and – at times, even get out of the way – like elephant "midwives," who surround the laboring mother in a circle but face outward as "look-outs," offering her privacy as well as protection.

Above all, the birth setting needs to be a place that feels safe. This may be a home or a hospital, or simply a preferred physical space. I think of one woman whom I interviewed for my doctoral research who gave birth in the way she wanted, with the midwife of her choice and the support of her partner. She remarked: "I have all my babies squatting in the hallway by the steps, in the darkest part of the house. It's just where I feel the safest." She shunned brightness and felt most comfortable giving birth at home in the dark without even the disturbance of moving to her bedroom where the midwife's equipment and birthing stool were waiting. She derived great satisfaction from determining what she wanted and being allowed to control her birthing environment.

It is the recommendation of the College of Midwives of Ontario that women's choice of birth place should be supported and honored. The evidence is clear in regard to the safety, cost-effectiveness, and optimal outcomes of planned home birth for healthy women with trained, well-equipped caregivers. The Canadian Association of Midwives (CAM) now recommends this birthplace for normal births, signaling a shift away from defending choice of birthplace. A similar shift is also evident in the current encouragement of breastfeeding. Ever careful not to offend, sensitive proponents of breastfeeding used to feel they should mutter "breast is best" *sotto voce*, rather than openly recommend it, even though there was much evidence for the superiority of breast milk. In addition, CAM's statement now acknowledges a much broader concept of safety than simply the physiological; all caregivers are expected to have an awareness of the cultural, social, personal, and emotional safety of laboring women and their families.

The publication of *Joyful Birth* is timely. The Ontario government's recent call for Birth Center proposals leads us to anticipate long-awaited midwife-led free-standing birthing centers. More women in Ontario will be able to choose conditions for a pleasurable birth from among the widest range of sites, whether at home, in a birth center or a hospital, in a birthing pool – or in a dark hallway.

As *Joyful Birth* so amply shows too, birth is a source of profound joy, not only for the woman but for all involved – the midwife or doula and other close participants. The woman's partner or friends may be there during the labor, so cool and rational at first, and then be deeply moved by the birth and sob openly, with deep feeling. Who can forget the moment when the five-year-old wants to put gloves on, and puts her head next to yours to help her mother catch the baby? Or when the grandmother kneels down on her one good knee and receives the placenta. Or those moments right after a birth, when the siblings tumble over the bed with wonder, seeking to grasp the baby's tiny hand, bringing little gifts. Having played a part as a caregiver, you step back and feel the privilege of witnessing these magic moments. And as you quietly move into the background, a profound happiness comes over you. These are impressions that last forever.

One of the most exciting bodies of research to emerge in recent decades speaks to the medical and psychosocial benefits of the continuous support and presence of a female caregiver at a woman's birth – a family member, friend, doula, midwife or doctor, whether or not this woman is a professional. With such continuous support come shorter labors, a decreased need for pain relief, lower cesarean rates, and higher APGAR scores for babies. And women feel greater satisfaction with their birthing experiences. Given these advantages, it would seem that the continuous support of another woman should be readily available, free of charge, to all birthing women. The regulation of fully funded midwives who provide primary care for women during the prenatal, birth, and postpartum periods in hospital, home or birthing center was a hard-won victory. The funding and regulation of the supportive presence of a doula for women would provide a valuable public service.

Joyful Birth details how all labor attendants might help women: with quiet presence, active listening, support and responsiveness, as well as (where appropriate) massage, eye contact, affirmation, breath and sound work, imagery, position changes, and intuitive preparatory emotional work. In doing so, this book acts in part as a primer of the rules, ethics, and *modus operandi* of the doula.

In my doctoral research, I found that women described their midwives as their ally and advocate, speaking repeatedly in terms of intimate relationships with them, and their responsive and caring support. They spoke glowingly as well of the business of midwifery, of the caregiving functions the midwife performs to meet the needs of clinical care and management according to prescribed guidelines and evidence-based practices. In this book, we see how the doula's role complements and supports that of the midwife. One doula referred to the arrival of the midwives as "gentle angels of the night."

However, a few of the stories told in *Joyful Birth* may serve as cautionary tales for caregivers, particularly midwives. Like all of us, midwives are subject to the pressures of work and life that may at times have unwanted and unintended effects. Some of the portrayals in *Joyful Birth* will be disturbing for midwives who would see themselves as responsive, flexible, and non-authoritarian. This book at times challenges midwives' self-definition as working to redefine birth both broadly within the health care system, and in the moment of each woman's individual birth, as an empowering and meaningful life experience.

There is much to be learned from the stories of these women and their doulas as care providers. There is deep value in self-reflection for midwives and all caregivers, and in attending to the possibilities of hierarchies of intimacy developing in birth settings with multiple care providers playing multiples roles. The narratives in this book might serve as valuable reminders to midwives, as well as all caregivers, to continue to cherish and nurture our passion for meeting the very diverse needs of women as best as we can.

According to the Centre for the Advancement of Interprofessional Education (CAIPE), "Interprofessional Education occurs when two or more professions learn with, from, and about each other to improve collaboration and the quality of care." Despite the significant differences in the scope of practice of the doula and the midwife, they have much in common. Collaborations occur and hierarchies diminish as caregivers work in partnership with the woman.

Through the stories of this book we are reminded that it is helpful for caretakers to avoid the pitfall of essentializing the birth experience: that is, building up a strongly held belief that a birth should fit a proscribed or ideal pattern – that the perfect birth is unmedicated, takes place at home, and is joyful, for instance. However, *what* happens around birth may not be as important as *how* it happens.

A birth that I particularly recall was one attended by Dr. Murray Enkin years ago. The baby was breech and many attempts had been made to turn the baby. Murray was open to a vaginal breech birth; however, the baby didn't descend. After much consultation with the birthing couple, a cesarean delivery was planned. What I especially remember was the fun and pleasure in the birthing room that night, centred around the new parents. Yes, there was disappointment that the birth wasn't a hoped-for vaginal birth, but there was sweetness there. Everyone associated with the event had brought their best, their most thoughtful selves, and then gratitude flowed.

We know that birth is not always joyful. Cynthia Gabriel's research on the experiences of some Russian women giving birth found that suffering was expected and embraced. For most women birthing in Canada, because of the ready availability of pain relief medication, the choice to experience birthing pain is voluntary. Pamela Klassen notes that there are many women who already suffer great pain in their particular socioeconomic contexts, for whom the experience of birthing pain may not be a privilege but an additional suffering. In addition, as Sheryl Nestel points out, some may romanticize midwifery and birthing practices in non-dominant cultures without understanding how patriarchal oppression, poverty and difficult working conditions actually affect the health and choices of childbearing women and their midwives.

The collection of stories in *Joyful Birth* is particularly welcome, given that it appears in the midst of a global crisis when the incidence of medical and surgical interventions for birth is increasing at an alarming rate. In many settings, induction of labor and epidurals are the norm and cesarean birth rates range from 30% to 70% with a corresponding rise in maternal morbidity. In under-resourced areas of the world, equitable access to adequate midwifery and obstetrical care is still not possible, and the United Nations Fifth Millennium Goal to reduce maternal mortality by three quarters has not yet reached its target. In some of my travels to developing countries, I have seen that efforts to improve infant and maternal mortality by moving births to institutionalized settings are in fact replicating the worst in Western maternity care; women give birth in crowded facilities, are separated from their family and loved ones, and birth alone in a dehumanized, assembly-line fashion.

Women bring multiple meanings to birth. Some of those meanings are expressed in the candid accounts of these chapters. Again, I congratulate Lisa Caron and Lisa Doran for gathering these stories and bringing this book to fruition. I invite you to immerse yourself in *Joyful Birth* and enjoy its wide variety of stories and experiences. They are testaments to the universality, yet individuality, of the birthing experience and illustrate just why each woman needs to be offered the care that respects and responds to her wishes.

Mary Sharpe, RM, MEd, PhD

Note: Sections of the Foreword have previously appeared in the author's PhD dissertation: "Intimate-Business: Woman-Midwife Relationships in Ontario, Canada."

Introduction

by Lisa Doran

JOYFUL EXPERIENCES OF BIRTH should not be underestimated. I am a story teller at heart and have been a doula since 1991. I have seen wonderful things and have learned incredible lessons "with woman" as a doula. I am also a naturopathic doctor and have specialized in reproductive endocrinology, obstetrics, and gynecology for most of my 15-year career. I teach the third-year course in Maternal Newborn Care at the Canadian College of Naturopathic Medicine in Toronto. Sharing the narrative experience of what I have learned with my clients, my patients, and my students is woven into my life. I could not begin to talk to women about birth without the use of cases from my naturopathic or doula practice.

When my teaching partner, Dr. Kirsten Perley, ND, and I took over the Maternal Newborn Care course, we felt it was very important to bring the course out of the textbook realm of obstetrical facts and figures and into the very real and exciting front-line clinical world of women's health and wellness. We decided to create the entire first lecture to focus on the importance of a woman's birth experience and why it is important to her future decision making, self-esteem, and even her mothering style.

As a physician and educator I advocate for a woman to make her own decisions for her pregnancy and birth. This will result in a more positive and empowering experience. Women who have a positive birth experience feel more confident in their new role as mother. They suffer less from postpartum depression, they breastfeed for longer periods of time, and they have an easier time responding to their infant's needs. Women who have positive birth experiences also communicate that they feel better bonded with their infants. Clearly, this has important effects on both mother and infant and on future child development and health. It is also exciting, as someone who works with women in the prenatal period, to know that if I can help women understand how their decision making during their pregnancy affects long-term health and wellness of both themselves and their children, then I can start to be more effective in helping women to implement long-term wellness-based lifestyle changes. Understanding this important piece of prenatal care has completely changed how I approach naturopathic care of the pregnant woman.

I spend considerable time educating these women about their pregnancy. For example, I am able to provide resources and simple practical tools for women so they can make decisions about stressors in their life. They learn the connection between experiencing every-day stress AND the resultant increased stress hormones. Stress experienced by the mother affects her baby profoundly and has subsequent long-term effects. Another great example is educating patients around common household environmental toxins in their cleaning solutions, their cosmetics, the plastics they use for cooking and food, and the long-term effects fetal exposure can have on attention and focus in children, on the future fertility of these children, and even on their immune responsiveness.

When Lisa Caron and I put out our call for authors for the first book in this series, *Bearing Witness: Childbirth Stories Told by Doulas,* we were delighted with all of the wonderful stories that we received discussing birth and women's experience of birth as they participated in the important work of being a doula and supporting women. As the book came together, one of the things that stood out in my mind was that many of the stories discussed how difficult it was for the doula to bear witness to some of the things that happen in birth – most especially in modern obstetrical practises. There were many stories that were difficult to read but as someone who had worked in the birth field for 20 years, I was not surprised by these stories. As a result of working on *Bearing Witness*, I learned two valuable things. Positive experiences of birth affect everyone involved – even those simply observing, and our narrative discussions of our experience of birth, either as mothers or as doulas, were extremely important learning tools for childbearing women.

I am in no way defining what a "joyful birth" is except to simply say that the mother conveys a positive experience. I have attended cesarean births that women reported as very positive and empowering, and I have attended home births that were not at all described with positive language. In 2006, I conducted an on-line survey of more than 400 women across North America asking questions about their birth experience: 77% of the women who had homebirths described their experience as positive, but only 36% of the women who had hospital births described their experience as positive; 84% of homebirthers described a positive immediate bonding period with their newborn babies whereas women who birthed in the hospital only 18% reported they were able to positively bond with their babies after the birth.

I would like to share two examples from the survey:

> My birth experience was wonderful, my son cut the cord, and my grandmother watched a baby being born for the very first time. There was such love and support in that room. The baby was beautiful. I find that the baby was born into lots of love. I think that having the baby born at home allowed me the special bonding time with the baby immediately after birth, there was no periods of separation.

Oh, it was very magical. I worked hard, but I really don't remember much. I just remember floating in the water and massaging my baby through my tummy and sleeping between rushes. I remember reaching down and pulling my own baby up to my chest and how time seemed to stand still and how everything was quiet. Hearing him cry out briefly and then look into my eyes was wonderful.

Here are two examples of a negative experience reported in the survey:

It was difficult to bond when I missed his first look around the room; he didn't open his eyes again for me for two days. I still mourn that lost time.

I still cry sometimes when I talk about his birth. Having another c-section was devastating. I have very few memories in the 24 hours after his birth. I don't remember holding him for the first time or nursing him for the first time.

This survey was fascinating because it confirmed for me that the choice of place of birth and the circle of care a woman chooses for her pregnancy was one of the greatest factors in achieving a positive or negative birth experience. This was interesting to me as when you speak to many young women about birth, their main concern is the pain. Clearly, this factor is managed by women who birth at home, and clearly the effective management of this factor in a hospital environment is not contributing to increased positive experiences.

I was fortunate enough to be relaxing and chatting one day with one of my mentors in birth, discussing the recent publication of *Bearing Witness,* when we came to the subject of positive birth experience reporting and the importance of the narrative story and learning. It was her assertion that the narrative story, one in which the author describes her experience and then perhaps discusses her processing of the experience, was an important teaching and learning tool. Reading stories about birth is important for women who are planning a pregnancy. Important to their decision making and their own education and information about the process, and important for those who work in birth so that they have the opportunity to experience many more situations in birth as well as understanding long term effects of decision making. She felt that *Bearing Witness* was an important contribution to the field because it used narrative voices exclusively. I was concerned that many of the stories in *Bearing Witness* discussed difficult issues for those who work in the birth field. Many of the issues and concerns they had were about modern obstetrical practises. It was at that point that the idea for a book that emphasized positive experience was born and today we have 40 voices bringing you *Joyful Birth*.

When you open this book there are many interesting things that flow out. One of the most interesting to me is the emphasis on midwifery-attended birth and homebirth. As for the percentage of the submissions we received for consideration for *Joyful Birth* – however the authors wanted to define "joyful" – the large majority were in the context of midwifery care or choices around home birth. I find this very exciting. I am an unabashed advocate for both midwifery care and home birth. I have had three midwifery attended homebirths of my own and have attended as a doula and a naturopathic doctor at hundreds of others. Midwives have such an important and vital role in the health of mothers and babies and play such a key role for those healthy decisions women make in their pregnancies that create an entire generation of healthier people. As more mothers, and those who assist them, begin to raise their voices and discuss joyful birth experiences, I think these voices will encourage women to explore options that they perhaps didn't realize they had. Or perhaps to opt out of some of our mainstream obstetrical practises that "medicalize" birth and instead empower mothers to make healthy decisions for themselves and their babies.

I received the following from a father after the homebirth of their first child:

Susan has grown stronger as a woman and has learned something about herself: that she is capable of doing anything!

She experienced the birthing process the way god/the universe/mother nature intended. And because of this, she learned something about herself and discovered a side of herself that she did not know before. She was truly conscious and present, she lost herself in the infinite moment. She awakened an innate intelligence and summoned a power that she didn't know she had.

She discovered a little bit more of who she really is. She learned to trust herself, trust her body, and to trust nature's way. This is the essence of life: to experience, to learn who you are, and self-discover. The Buddhists talk of "suffering" in order to reach enlightenment. Susan "suffered" through the birth experience, and she was enlightened with a new understanding of herself and a new life: James William. He was sent to teach us, to enlighten and illuminate our lives. Susan and I will nurture him as he nurtures us!

I am hoping you enjoy reading *Joyful Birth* and that the lessons within speak to your heart.

Lisa Doran, BSc, ND

Ruby and the Placenta

by Carla Tonelli

THERE'S A PLACENTA IN MY FREEZER.

It was mine and Ruby's for 9 months, or 42 weeks and 2 days, if you were counting. Of course, I was. And my midwives. And the ultrasound people at the hospital because if you're over 42 weeks the baby's fluid starts to dry up and you can run into problems.

Our placenta is here because Ruby was born at home, in our little house, on our one-way street in High Park, Toronto. Bylaws forbid throwing human organs in the garbage (go figure!). We would like to bury it in the backyard, but the ground is still frozen so we are waiting for spring.

Ruby was late by 16 days. She weighed 7 lbs 2 oz and her skin was a little dry and old man-ish, but otherwise perfect – a perfect final addition to our family.

Her birth was messy, in my opinion, but not having witnessed many births my points of reference are few. Was it joyous? Oh yes.

She was my third baby, second born at home, first born here on purpose. Home births strike fear into the boomer generation but resonated loud and happily with me.

It's my bedsheets, which feel and smell the way I like. It's familiar art on the wall. The same bathroom I use every day down the hall. My lavender essential oil (which, for the record, does not trigger labor – I tried).

There are no stirrups at the foot of my bed. No parade of nurses changing guard, coming in to check my cervix's dilation.

Husband Gregor even had the liberty to make a beef stew in an attempt to keep my iron levels up (I'm borderline anemic). A team of vegetarian midwives in the house and we're smelling it up with stew – but whatever, it was an aroma of pure love so all anyone could say was, "What an amazing husband."

And he was amazing.

Our setup wasn't completely without modern medical advancements. We were prepared for anything, including being told to get in a car and get to a hospital, if it had come to that. We even had gas in the car.

So our bedroom was transformed into a traveling medical clinic in disguise, with the blue pads and sterilized equipment laid out on our dresser but mugs of tea and novels also strewn about.

I had an IV poking into my left hand because I was strep B positive and that could be bad for the baby if you don't pump an antibiotic into your system ahead of delivery. But my incredible chief midwife Becky (she'd never call herself a chief but I would) was also a nurse in a past life and was able to tee all that up for me.

So for eight hours I labored, we labored. We were going hard on the natural induction methods – sweeping membranes, walking, spicy food, sex, drinking castor oil (which has the consistency of runny Jell-O if you mix it with juice). So when the contractions finally started we were all relieved we wouldn't have to go anywhere near triage.

My memories are fragments, like a shattered mirror. But some things are closer to the surface.

I had a really hard time in phase two, the pushing, because it hurt hurt hurt. Sylvia Plath described it as "the black" in her journal account of the home birth of her son Nicholas. Black works for me; I can understand black.

Pain is really hard to nail down in words. Imagine putting your midsection in a vice, and turning that lever. Or having a watermelon slamming down on your rectum (from the inside). It is not like the flu, and it is not like a headache. Horrible diarrhea cramps are getting closer, but it is so intense all you can do is writhe. And breathe. And get mad at people for telling you to breathe.

At about the seventh hour, I was so tired. I wanted to go to sleep and try again in the morning. (It was 1:00 a.m). Someone suggested the nitrous oxide I'd requested days before, and I went for it. I regretted not asking for it sooner.

I was drowning in a rocky, stormy sea, and someone threw me a buoy. I could stop gasping for air for 10 seconds and float away to a happy place. They say it "takes the edge off" but what it does is give a reprieve from having your insides put in a blender.

I could relax. I could stop tensing up, like a flinch before a blow, and ease up enough for Ruby to know it was safe to come out.

I could hold Gregor's hand and look into his eyes and tell him how I love him with every fiber of my being and he could say "Me too." Like a city was crumbling around us and we didn't care. Midwives doing their thing, patient angels of the night. And us in our own world.

At this point, the fun really began to start. Becky finally convinced me to try the medieval torture device of a birthing stool (my description, not hers). I hated that thing. It was like a magnet sucking a cannonball through my bowels.

But soon enough, Ruby crowned. Becky was right.

I stood for this part, leaning on whoever was closest, screaming and gasping and bearing down as they say like there was no tomorrow.

I think probably the most amazing thing about childbirth, the most joyous, is just when you think you're about to die, you don't.

All that pain just stops.

From 60 to 0.

But the horrible stretching and tearing of your most sensitive parts is over, just like a snap of your fingers. And something slimy and slithery slides out of your body (watch out – it's fast!), and there's a huge bumpy long cord still coming out of you and it's so gross but it's so beautiful and you're done done done and there's a PERSON there, who wasn't there a minute ago, and she looks just like you, or is it your husband, and your midwife is beaming and trying not to drop her but she's so slippery and then there she is on your chest starting to murmur and open her eyes and she has these little fists that have never felt air before and they are up by her ears that have never heard our noises before and everything is fresh and new and the most amazing miracle, ever, anywhere, in any reality, has just happened. Here in your own little bedroom.

And there are no words.

There is elation and pride and I am on another planet. Someone is kissing my tears away.

Hello, girl.

I am meeting my baby.

It didn't matter that I was bruised and torn and would need an extra 30 minutes of stitching, or that no one had the aerosol numbing agent for a very big needle like I'd heard about in California.

It was over, it was beginning, and she was here.

There were plenty more things that happened that night. The delivery of the placenta, for one. But when you have a 5-minute-old baby on your breast nothing else seems to matter.

What an absolute, unequivocal honor to be the one in the middle keeping the chain of life going.

I do believe if you push yourself you can accomplish amazing things.

Our babies are the proof.

The Most Perfect Birth in the Wild West

by Hilary Monk

IT HAD TO BE THE MOST UNPRE-
dictable, most wonderful birth I'd seen for a long while. I was
interning at a 'birth house' in Texas – make sure you say that with
just the right kind of long, drawn-out drawl – to get exposure to a
different style of midwifery, and to different kinds of clients than
I'd be likely to meet in the predominantly middle-class, over-edu-
cated urban demographic of my practice.

This house was home to a number of very talented, very devoted
midwives who, although they were happy to provide care to anyone
who showed up, were known in the neighborhood as Christian midwives. So, of course, a lot of their clientele came from the far right,
with a distinct evangelical bent, and were seeking spirit-led midwives.
They relied on their midwives to incorporate in their tool boxes, along
with rigorous standardized medical training and all the usual techno-
gadgets, a deep faith in the mercy and creativity of God in the birth
process. I attended more than a few births with a crowd of women
praying aloud, hour after hour, and then giving thanks with loud
weeping, clapping, and crying of 'Hallelujah!' once their new little con-
gregational member arrived for his or her dedication to the Lord.

Consequently, the image you might have of typical clients there would be way off the mark for this one particular couple. Each of them were singular, unprecedented in my experience. They were a strangely matched pair of folks: she was very tall, naturally blonde-as-blonde-could-be, who, despite the full bloom of her fourth pregnancy, striding into the clinic in her Stetson, riding boots and full swing skirt, looked as close as a real human could come to being the cowgirl version of Barbie; her partner was a behemoth of a man, with a furrowed brow and heavy beard, tattooed on each finger and elsewhere, who wore a denim vest with rip-marks on the cloth where what could once have been gang colors had been torn off. They'd come to the clinic, announced well ahead of time by the loud *blat-blat* of a fully loaded Harley Davidson, and I peeked out the lacy curtains of the main reception to watch her swing her great long legs off the back of the bike, and the two of them blow in like a kind of raucous tornado for their appointment.

Her baby was due around Christmas time, and this one evening they came into the clinic to drop off a huge turkey with all the fixings, and specific instructions to make sure that anybody coming to the clinic who needed something to eat and maybe had some kind of trouble getting or paying for it could have as much as they like. (They'd seen that once in a while this was a problem, sometimes with a Mexican woman or sometimes with a 15-year-old mom-to-be, who'd get left for a day or two at the clinic to give birth without anything to eat and no money.)

During our meetings, I'd learned about their lives. They were itinerant preachers, travelling from place to place, looking for homeless kids and other needy folks on the street, to bring them the Good Word and set them back onto a path of righteousness and happiness any way they could. The pamphlet they handed out recounted his tale of having been on death row for 23 years for a murder committed when he was 'astray' during his teen years. This had been no joke, for in Texas, death row was the real thing. During his time in jail, he'd been brought to the Lord, and had become a sincere follower of Jesus, without any thought of possible reprieve except for a spiritual salvation. Suddenly, word came down from out of the blue from the governor, and he found himself released with a full pardon, at the age of 40 never having conducted an adult life anywhere but in prison. He told it that God had sent him this beautiful lady to help him to create his Ministry and, much to his shock, to bring a new lamb to the flock.

Mid-morning, Roxie, my co-midwife, and I got a phone call that her waters had broken, and would it be all right if she came over, even though it was still pretty early. Of course, I said, we'd be delighted to get ready to receive her any time. We did our usual rushing around of making sure there were enough other midwives to cover the clinic appointments should she call us upstairs to attend her for any length of time, and setting up all the equipment for the birth in the prettiest of the birthing rooms. It was called the Summer room, and was just so sweetly appointed, with a beautiful antique walnut suite of furnishings, and cool green and warm pink fabrics swathed here and there to give it a fresh garden feel. Once the receiving blankets were all set to warm in the heating pads, back we went downstairs.

Soon enough, we heard the roar of the bike coming up the drive, and I was thinking, 'Man! What a way for a laboring lady to travel!' They came on in, and we filled out the papers and took her vitals and listened to the baby's heartbeat and so on while watching her carefully for any signs of pain or imminent delivery. During these rituals, she mentioned that some friends of theirs would come for support during labor, which was all fine by us. He was looking a little piqued, a little pale, and I thought this whole thing, now that it was down to the line, was maybe a bit too much for him. But his lovely lady was keeping his spirits up by being ever so affectionate with him and reassuring him that she was "Fine, jes' fine. No reason to worry 'tall honey."

I am sure the support their friends would provide would be for him as she seemed not to need a thing. In fact, neither I nor Roxie could see any indication that she was in labor, no grimacing, no unusual breathing, no clutching of her stomach or groaning, not even that strange light that comes into some women's eyes as their bodies rearrange hormone levels to allow for the birth. During the whole course of events, Roxie and I would signal to one another, lifting our eyebrows as if to say silently, "So? What do you think? I haven't a clue." Because her waters were broken and the babe's heart sounded right as rain, there was no need to do any poking about internally to determine progress until something indicated a need for it, or she asked.

The afternoon progressed, and sure enough their friends arrived – a whole cavalcade of motorcycles in a procession to our front door. As the clinic day drew to a close, I am sure the other clients were just as happy to get out of there, as what looked to become quite a party began to take shape. Their support team consisted of a number of burly men with bare, muscled arms sporting all kinds of tattoos and raw jewelry, and a couple brought along their women. These ladies, despite appearances to the contrary, did what all women do. They disappeared into the kitchen, along with our client, to prepare snacks and goodies for the guys, who sat about joking and teasing and reminiscing when one or the other had had a kid.

They'd brought along a video to pass the time, Whoopi Goldberg in *Sister Act*. While this was playing, aside from listening to the babe every so often, Roxie and I made ourselves scarce. Still our client was not displaying any labor signs. Instead, after laughing her way through most of the film perched easily on the arm of her husband's chair, she leaped up, ambled into the kitchen, made the biggest triple-decker turkey sandwich I've ever seen, and wolfed it down. Then, vigorously brushing her hands together to get rid of any residual crumbs, she sauntered back into the main room and announced, "I think we'll go upstairs now and have us a baby!"

Roxie and I shot astonished looks at one another, but, obediently, we followed her husband up to the birth room, all three of us trotting along behind her like a line of ducklings behind mother. Once in the room, we were ready to do all the usual things as she proceeded to remove her panties without the slightest ruffle or hesitation. But we'd barely got our gloves on, when she made her way to the high four-poster bed, clambered right up and lay on her side, holding one of those long legs way up and out of the way, knee to her chest. She looked over her shoulder at her husband and, giving him a huge, bright smile, with a gentle grunt, bore down – once, hard.

Out popped two little hands! She looked down at them, and laughed and said, "Oh look! She's praisin' the Lord already!" We were scrambling to help her receive the child, and I was trying not to laugh too hard, because it was tough to see through my tears. Sure enough, with her next push out came this gorgeous doll of a little girl, pink and wiggly, doing all the things a brand-new person does to show the world how ready she is to take it on. Still smiling from ear to ear, before she even touched the child herself, she said huskily to her husband, "Take her darlin' and show her to the Lord."

Now he had been watching this event, hanging onto his amazing wife's arm, his face getting redder and redder behind the great bush of beard, and his eyes getting wider and wider. As the little one was born, the tears welled over and ran down his face. At his wife's invitation, he gathered the baby up, so, so tenderly, his big hands shaking with emotion, lifted her high towards heaven, and he called out in a quavering voice full of awe and gratitude, "Thank you, Lord. Thank you, Jesus. Here's our baby, and she's yours."

From this point, things returned to normal – the placenta was delivered, she had not torn a bit, the baby was perfect. The friends whooped with glee at the news and toasted the couple before quietly taking turns going upstairs to meet the baby and wish them all well. We left the new family with the baby latched on contentedly at her mother's breast, and the father cradling them both in his huge embrace. It took a fair bit for Roxie and I to come down from this happy occasion. We went on to laugh uproariously at how she'd taken us by surprise, and at what had transpired, but I know that it was something truly special for us all.

♀ Technology of Cloth

by Julei Busch

Colloidal muscles flow with power,
overcoming body neuroses imposed
by a puritanical pathologizing of ecstasy.
Generations of women bound
by the technologies of touch and cloth
have imprinted birth as beautiful.
No shit-shocked liabilities in the house of rapture
where mammalian birth needs overcome fears of little death.

It is simply un-common sense to ignore
the bewildering congress of insurances
cackling grim fearful tales from monkey minds in stark cold rooms.
Rather, bring laughter and compassion to soothe the floating head
duality away.
Revealing the multilingual sphincter law, wiser hearts prevail.
With vision stretching beyond the birth gate,
amidst prayers for large openings and hollows,
amidst giggles and praise for functions even Emily Post could not
contain,
our collective grandmothers whisper:
"Breath deep and draw strength from all mothers before you.
Sing the uterus song set to a placental bass beat."

Not a witch burns here
where hands are placed with care,
as tidal forces wash away a river of denial.
Surrendering to the embrace of a rebozo,
to the sweet kiss of loving kindness,
we embody sovereignty and birth a new community.

Authors Note: This poem gestated awhile, for some months in fact, in the post-conference bliss of the potent phrases of a fearless woman, an outspoken midwife, a learned and powerful agent of change. This humble offering is dedicated to Ina May Gaskin. Thank you for your passion, persistence, and sheer stubborn determination to speak about the joy of birth often, and to all those who need to hear it.

Birth By Hand

by Beth Murch

FOR AS LONG AS I CAN REMEMBER, I have been a healer. I was aware that I stood with a foot in two very different worlds – the reality of the physical, where gravity's existence is made manifest by a falling apple and where a hand can trace the origin of that fruit by caressing the furrowed bark of a tree, and that of the other, a place of shadow and silver.

I knew from a very young age that our plane of verisimilitude was draped in a misty veil of an ethereal realm not unlike when my sister and I would wrap each other in our mother's window sheers, pretending to be brides. I learned quickly that I could vicariously experience the emotions of others, even when they did not tell me how they were feeling and that by opening my heart to the whispers of the Universe, I was able to harness what Elizabeth Cunningham, author of *The Maeve Chronicles*, aptly calls "the fire of the stars": an energy that came from that place beyond planets that circumnavigate the sun, beyond the inky blackness of space, beyond the jagged edges of stars that helped me to sense where a person's body or spirit needed repair and emanated as healing light from my ājñā, my heart and my hands.

I can recall being six or seven years old, and bending over my mother, who was stretched out on the floor before me, and using this capacity to identify where there was pain in her back, hips, and legs and then massaging her. "How do you know where to rub?" she asked me, her speech slurred with relaxation. "I just do," I replied, secretly both surprised and pleased at this gift that I could neither explain nor truly appreciate as an untrained young girl.

I do not consider myself to be someone who is well-schooled in healing; I have read books, taken classes in Reiki, explored concepts of divine intervention through ritualistic practice, and earned three university degrees, but I know from studying with masters infinitely more learned and attuned than I could ever hope to be, that I truly have little knowledge. I have made mistakes: sipped energy from those around me without their permission, conducted sessions of healing where I was not invited, and allowed myself to physically and emotionally decay by failing to construct a permeable membrane that would protect my physical and mental stability by preventing situations and folks who might consciously or unconsciously extract my intercession. In the green pasture where the thoroughbreds of shamans, seers, mystics, witches, priests, and preachers graze on stems and leaves, I am but a colt, wobbling on my gangly legs, simply attempting to walk without falling.

As a doula, I rely upon my abilities to heal. I open myself to that Other Realm and allow it to guide me in my work, letting it lead me when it comes to helping my clients. Alas, there are no special effects – there are no bolts of lightning, no earthquakes, no levitations, and no theme music – simply a pricking of my intuition that leads me to think about whether a laboring mother needs my hands on her, if her partner needs something to eat, or if a baby is posterior. At a mama's request, I might use reflexology, Reiki, homeopathy, prayer, or meditation to help her to be comfortable and to allow herself to be guided by her rushes, but I do not make medical predictions, I do not dispute the amazing abilities of "hard science," and I do not invoke powers that make people uncomfortable (for example, some faith groups are strongly uncomfortable with energy healing and I am respectful of that). I allow myself to be a vessel, and I simply try to pour out what is needed whether it is advice, reassurance, a hand to hold, pictures taken, placentas encapsulated, silent companionship or encouragement to breastfeed.

There is so much power in the room where a woman births. She stands at the door between Life and Death and a soul from the Other Side is called down. Labor tests her very mettle, challenging what she knows to be true, asking her to go into a place within herself that may be unfamiliar, and wearing at her physical stamina. The baby who emerges is a love letter from that realm that we cannot understand – the culmination of ancestors, rich earth and helixes, born into the fingerprints and destiny that it has chosen for itself long before it took root in its mother's womb. I am always in awe of the dance that takes place as it always has, as it always will, always as it needs to be.

During the summer of 2011, I was present at a woman's labor in a way that I had never been before and it truly allowed me to comprehend not just the incredible awesome power of birthing women, but also the privilege I have in being a doula and a healer.

I was hired by a couple to attend the birth of their second baby. I had been their doula at their first birth, a home waterbirth three years before, and it was a delight to be catching up and making plans for this new life joining us. Their requests were very simple: Papa did not want to cut the cord or touch the baby until it was born and Mama wanted the midwives to carry extra Pitocin with them in order to avoid a hemorrhage, which she experienced along with some nasty tearing with her first delivery. Mama had a short labor, so we knew that the likelihood of this birth progressing quickly was high. I kept my doula kit packed and ready to go at a moment's notice.

The call came early in the evening, around dinnertime.

"I'm feeling *something*," Mama said. "It could be gas or it could be labor."

"Okie-dokie," I said, with a sense that this was the beginning of labor.

About half an hour or forty-five minutes later, Papa called me. I heard heavy breathing in the background. "Yeah ... we're going to need you to come on over now," he said. His nervous excitement made his voice quiver.

I took a taxi over to my clients' house and arrived within the hour. I knocked on the door and almost immediately Papa opened it for me. Mama was standing in the dining room, in front of the birth tub, wearing a t-shirt and panties. Her feet were planted wide apart and she was looking down at the floor.

"My water just broke!" she exclaimed. "Like, just as you knocked on the door, my water broke!"

"Good!" I said. "That means things are coming along nicely! Were the fluids clear?"

"We're not quite sure. They seemed clear, but there was a piece of something brown in them that could have been meconium, I'm not sure. We wiped it up already."

Suddenly, she grabbed her round, taut belly and moaned, "Here we go!"

She leaned on me as she swayed through her contraction, her hips making the circle for infinity, the same movement women have done since the beginning of time as they birthed their babies in thickets and caves, tents and wagons, feather beds and hospital rooms. I stayed silent, listening, trying to read the language of her body.

She is close, I thought.

"They're stronger now," Mama said.

"Yes, when your water breaks, things get a lot more intense. Did you call the midwives?"

"Right when we called you," Papa said, pacing back and forth. "They said they would be here soon."

"Here's another one!" Mama said, hissing out air through clenched teeth. We rocked together and I felt the plate tectonics taking place within her: her pelvis spreading open, her ligaments stretching, the baby's head tucking under the pubic bone. As her rush concluded, she gave a little grunt.

"I kind of felt 'pushy' with that one."

"Oh, really?" I asked, not entirely surprised. "That's okay. We knew this labor would go faster than your first one. The midwives will be here soon."

"What should we do?" Papa asked, clearly anxious.

"Fill up the birth tub!" Mama snapped, clearly about to have another contraction.

"That's a good idea," I agreed. "It's definitely not too soon to start doing that."

Papa rushed about, attaching the hose to the kitchen sink and turning on taps.

"Mmmmm …. uhhh … ohhhhh…." moaned Mama, shifting her weight from side to side. The palms of my hands, which were around her waist, started to burn with the ferocity of her labor, and I noticed the energy exchange taking place between Mama and I was fervid. My hands always tingle when a baby is being born, and as I stood there, still in my shoes, I started to have a sneaking suspicion that the midwives' arrival was going to be a photo finish with the baby's. The perimeters between worlds were dissolving, melting away to allow this child a passage through one realm into another.

"I could definitely push," Mama said. "Oh yes. I'm feeling pressure."

"Let's get you on your hands and knees," I said. "Sometimes, that slows things down a little bit."

I walked Mama into the living room and she knelt down in front of the couch, resting her forehead on the seat. I squatted beside her and rubbed her back. I heard her breath become jagged and she began to sob.

"Ican'thavethebabynowthemidwifeisn'thereandIwanthertobe-hereit'stoosoontoosoonohohoh" she cried in one terribly long sentence, her tears making dark marks on the sofa.

At that moment, the middle of what I lovingly refer to as a woman's "pre-baby freak out" – I realized that I was going to be playing more than one role at this labor. I had always known that at least once in my doula career, there would be a time where a baby came before the midwife arrived or before the mother got to the hospital. That time was now.

"Oh, Honey, it's okay! Your baby is ready to be born, and that's a good thing! When labors are this fast, it's usually because everything is going just fine. I know what to do. You are safe and your baby is safe. Don't cry! It's your baby's birthday! This is a happy moment!"

A pressure wave rose up again from deep inside of Mama and as I watched it crest, I observed her thighs shaking and the way her body strained.

"Are you pushing?" I asked, even though I knew the answer already.

"Mmmhmm." Mama breathed.

"Is it all right if I just take a look?" I asked.

I remember Mama saying yes, and I remember the way the dark cotton felt as I hooked my fingers around the waistband of her underwear and pulled them down. I instantly smelled it: the feral odor of birth. It is an unmistakable perfume: the tang of metallic blood, the sweet notes of amniotic fluid, the musk of vaginal secretions, the whiff of sweat, and the pungent aroma of feces. This is what they don't tell you in doula school, that parturition has a scent, that you will carry that scent in your clothes and in your hair, that you will love the raw perfume of woman's most private parts.

I looked down between Mama's legs expecting to see a slight part in her labia as her body moved the baby down with the contractions. Instead, I saw an egg-sized portion of fetal scalp.

"IS THAT THE BABY?" Papa shouted from the doorway to the living room, incredulously.

"Yes, that's your baby," I replied, keeping my voice even and calm, even though my heart was skipping a few beats. "Do you have any towels or blankets?"

"Which should I get? Towels or blankets?"

I watched the bit of head withdraw slightly into the vagina and then ease out a fraction more.

"I don't think it matters," I responded, hoping not to sound too snippy. "Just something nice and warm to wrap the baby in. Oh! And a bowl! Get a bowl for the placenta."

I turned to Mama and put my hand upon her shoulder.

"Your baby is right there. I can see part of the head."

I prayed that Goddess would bless my hands and that the wisdom of all the healer women who had come before me would be with me that night.

I narrated the events unfolding before me to the pale man standing at the threshold of the room and to the strong woman working hard before me.

"Your baby's forehead is out. Look! I see little ears! Aww. Look at the little eyes."

The baby's head burst forth from between the petals of Mama's labia like a flower blooms on a warm spring morning and came to rest in my cupped hands. Kneeling on the floor, holding that tiny noggin in my outstretched hands, with the holy altar of the yoni before me, I felt engaged in the purest form of worship possible. For a moment, I felt a divine connection that transcended time and space; a force of love more powerful than anything anyone could ever imagine, a fierce potency that blazed through my body like a wildfire. I was bearing witness to a miracle – a miracle that may happen hundreds of times a day, all across the world, but a miracle no less.

I called upon my healing power to speak to the baby without opening my mouth.

Okay, Baby – your job now is to rotate so that your shoulders are born.

I know, she replied. I've done this before.

And so, the baby gave a little wriggle and turned towards the left. I tucked my index finger in its armpit and the shoulders were quickly born. With a final push, a beautiful baby girl slide out into the world, with a tsunami of amniotic fluid and blood following behind her, splashing on the laminate flooring. I clasped the slippery child to my chest, smearing creamy vernix across my shirt, and I watched as mucus poured from her nose and mouth. She took a deep breath and gave a soft little cry and then moved her limbs hesitantly.

I had Papa help Mama stand up and then passed the baby to her, through her legs, still attached to the umbilical cord. I placed a towel over the baby and rubbed her a bit, more in the interest of pinking her up than getting her clean. She was breathing just fine – she was simply a peaceful baby who was more interested in sniffing and licking her mother and looking around than crying. Mama sang the same Pagan welcoming song that she sang to her new daughter's big sister when she was born, and I had Papa take some pictures.

By the time the midwives arrived, Mama was nursing and drinking some juice, and Papa was making phone calls to family members to let them know that the baby was born. Both the midwives kept asking me if I was okay, as if they thought I might be in shock. I wish I had the words to tell them that I was better than okay, I was feeling the best I have ever felt in my entire life! My heart was filled with so much joy that I felt like I was going to float away into the atmosphere like a helium balloon.

For all our worries about hemorrhaging, Mama did just fine. She received two shots of Pitocin and the placenta was delivered with ease. She only had a skid mark – no tearing, which was a relief to both of us. Papa was still adamant that he did not want to cut the umbilical cord, so he and Mama graciously allowed me to do it myself. As I used the scissors, I said a blessing:

"Blessed are You, Goddess our Mother, who creates us and sustains us and allowed us to reach this occasion. Amen."

After tidying up and making sure everyone was comfy, I went home. I flopped on the couch and looked at myself. My clothes were covered in birth fluids. My hair was damp with sweat. My hands … my hands were steady, strong, and charged with the healing power of all the wise women who had come before me, who had stood with one foot in the physical world and one foot in the ethereal world to call down souls.

♀ Endure

by Keshia Kamphuis

You are ten moons of mystery,
a thousand hours of miracle unfolding;
Where living roots cradle your beginning
in a cosmic tide of abundant blessing.
In this sanctuary of becoming you wait
for the whisper of tomorrow's longing.

She is the wisdom of every woman,
a thousand years of birth unfolding;
Where an ancient prose tells of growing curves,
innate in its knowing, timeless in its enduring.
It is this rhythm that keeps count and calls forth:
the moment is now.

In this hour, surrendering moans fill this place
and hands clutch in steadfast determination;
Where exhales ache and hopeful words praise,
lifting spirits to greater possibilities.
These our gifts to a warrior Mother
in plight to meet her promised child.

One thread weaves this moment's tapestry,
joining the stories of our witnessing;
Where Life keeps vigil in candle cast shadows
as gentle passages transform to light.
Here final sighs meet joyful cries of breath,
proclaiming Life, declaring Being.

Universal Love manifest in your life,
a sacred gift of conceiving and creating.
Where whispers affirm this hour's life,
our tears of beholding, these hands of blessing;
To share this Journey our humble offering –
bringing all that we can, being all that we are.

Authors Note: Inspired by bearing witness to the birth of my nephew, Dante Campos-Kamphuis. Dante means enduring or lasting. May every woman find what it is to endure in this great journey of motherhood.

Emma and Arish

by Kerry Grier

CHANCE IS A FINE THING. IF I HADN'T been geographically challenged I would not have accepted the trek out to Brampton to teach Arish and Emma. I was new to Toronto and hadn't yet realized that time and distance calculations are meaningless when it comes to roadwork and traffic. I am so happy I didn't miss the chance to meet this lovely family and now regularly travel farther afield.

Arish and Emma are a young professional couple living in an immaculate, spacious home. Everything about them told me that they are on top of things, and the impending arrival of their baby was the icing on the cake.

I knew from the first HypnoBirthing session that both Arish and Emma were ideal candidates. One of the many pleasures of my work as a prenatal and HypnoBirthing instructor is the wonderful people I come into contact with. I feel privileged to be a part of their birth journeys. Arish and Emma were one such example. Emma relaxed quickly and totally under hypnosis, and Arish was very supportive and enjoyed the relaxation too.

They had done their research and knew that a natural,

unmedicated birth was their goal. Emma was the product of a natural birth and, having grown up in Kenya, had experienced nothing but natural births in her entourage. Her birth meter was set to "normal and uneventful" barring special circumstances.

The HypnoBirthing classes progressed well, and each week I was delighted to see Emma blossoming more and more and Arish's excitement at impending fatherhood mounting.

Alas, all too soon, we had completed the training and it was time to part ways. I always empathize with mother birds at this point in the moments before they launch their babies from the nest. Emma and Arish were ready though. They were primed to bring their baby into the world in the calm and nurturing way we had envisaged together. They listened to their practice CD regularly and had even recorded one of our sessions to use up until the birth.

During the last class, they asked if I would come back to teach baby care and breast feeding basics and also if I would consider being their birth doula. I agreed to teach baby care and breast feeding, but much as I wanted to be there for the birth, I did not want to over-promise. They would be going to a hospital farther from my home than I usually venture, and Emma had chosen 5 hours as the length of her labor and tightening as the sensation of her surges. My concern was, as with many HypnoBirthing mothers, she may not realize she was in active labor until it was almost over, and although she would get to the hospital in time, I may not. We decided to play it by ear.

Shortly after Emma reached 40 weeks, on a crisp early summer morning, Arish called me. He wanted to know if I thought Emma was in labor – she was experiencing a "tightening sensation" fairly regularly, but it was not painful. She was in the shower and felt fine. I said I would take my small daughters home and see them soon. Within 20 minutes I texted to say "On my way to you," which was autocorrected to say "On my way to tornado" – hardly a message you want to get from your HypnoBirthing instructor and doula!

What followed could not be further from a tornado. The gradual unfolding of events like so many petals unfurling was a joy.

Emma was calm and excited about the imminent arrival of her baby. She had bloody show just after I arrived, and we started to time the surges. Arish, an APP designer, had come across an APP to do this and we took it in turns timing. We watched Dr. Harvey Karp's "Happiest Baby on the Block" DVD, and I smiled to myself thinking that all the ingredients were there for this little baby to be the happiest on the block indeed! A loving family, a calm and nurturing birth and an extended family bursting with anticipation to love this small person. Emma was experiencing tightening sensations, which were clearly present but not painful. Her main discomfort was that she was tired, having had a fitful night the night before. Arish was tired, too, as was Emma's mother.

Everyone found a comfy spot and I took them into a relaxation hypnosis. Within minutes the house was in silence with everyone fast asleep. I tiptoed into the kitchen and read my book while they all caught up with some much needed sleep. One theory I have heard is that 15 minutes in the Alpha state of brainwaves, such as is experienced under hypnosis, is the equivalent of an hour's sleep. Judging by how refreshed everyone was after an hour's rest, I think there is truth to this.

The surges were by now every six minutes, and Emma was showing no inclination to head to the hospital a good 40 minute drive away. She was hungry and her mother had prepared a wonderful vegetarian lunch. We ate and then I announced that I am not a midwife or an obstetrician so we needed to head for the hospital. Emma looked so comfortable I think she would have stayed exactly where she was, given the choice! A part of her I think did not believe that this could be labor.

In the car on the way to the hospital the surges picked up in frequency and intensity. We used a trigger word to help her relax, but I think the restricted movement was making some of the surges uncomfortable.

Arish's mother and brother had followed us to the hospital and were anxiously waiting in the family room. We sent them home to wait for news. It is important for a HypnoBirthing mother to be able to completely relax and not feel under any pressure to give constant updates.

Emma is not a fan of hospitals but within minutes she and Arish had unpacked things from home. Soon music was playing and candles were burning, which later proved to be a no no. Last but not least, a picture of their guru.

I know very little about the Hindu religion and asked them to tell me a bit about it. The overriding quality is kindness to fellow people and creatures. It is no surprise then that they were choosing such a peaceful entry into the world for their baby.

The surges were effective and picking up. Emma paced and rocked her way through them looking like she had stepped out of a fashion magazine. She was wearing a turquoise kaftan her mother had brought from Kenya, which offset her thick glossy hair and luminous skin. Birthing mothers have such a beauty about them, and Emma was positively glowing.

We used some trigger words to relax Emma through her surges and also used some less conventional methods! As a surprise for Emma, some weeks earlier, Arish had taken them to a Laughing Yoga weekend. I asked them to demonstrate, knowing that the oxytocin produced when we laugh does wonders to speed up labor. They stood and looked at each other, palms upwards and would make a statement and sweeping motion followed by laughter that went something like this:

"I am happy!" (sweeping motion downwards with hands then laughter, which at first sounded forced but within seconds was genuine laughter).

This would then be answered by the other along these lines:

"I am courageous!"
Downward sweep ... Ha ha ha!

Try it. I dare you! It makes you feel like a million bucks!

I had also come armed with a coloring book I had picked up at the ROM featuring infuriatingly detailed Indian tapestries. I handed it to Emma and said that the only thing she had to worry about was coloring in one of those pictures. She immediately got started and soon was lost in concentration. She has that picture still.

Every three to four minutes a surge would wash through her, she would pause, and Arish would stand up and say: "I am Amazing!" sweep, "Ha! Ha! Ha!" and Emma would laugh.

We also used one of her relaxation triggers. These included placing a hand on her shoulder, a special word, her birth color, and imagining a quiet place in nature.

We also used light touch massage to confuse her neural pathways and steer them away from any sensations of pain.

As the surges grew more intense, we started to count our way through some of them. Counting to ten while pressing firmly on her thighs seemed to help a lot, and to make it more complicated, we counted in as many languages as the three of us could think up. Emma and Arish clocked up about six languages between them, and I added another three or four. When we ran out of our own languages, we prevailed upon Eva, the lovely Nigerian nurse, to step in with her own Igbo.

We had discussed a very detailed birth plan and the hospital stuck to it to the letter. The staff was wonderfully supportive of HypnoBirthing, despite being unfamiliar with it, and left us to our own devices. Internal examinations were few and far between, lights were dimmed, and we had very few interruptions.

Upon admission Eva had examined Emma and said she was at 3 centimeters. We did not concern ourselves overly with measurements because we knew that Emma was doing wonderfully and everything was just as it should be.

Soon Emma decided to take a bath and found the jets to be very soothing. She lay in the tub, with us periodically adding more hot water, for about an hour. During this time she was very centerd and in a state of complete relaxation. Whenever she had a particularly strong surge, she would smile and say, "I can do this, I am doing this." And doing it she was.

She was awakened from her revery by what turned out to be her baby ready to be born. Unfortunately, a water birth was not an option so we helped her onto the bed. She was at 10 centimeters.

An obstetrician gave her the go-ahead to push, and even though this is not part of HypnoBirthing, she decided to push with all her might. She was getting tired and wanted to meet her baby.

Her petite frame belied a strength that took us all by surprise and she was a champion pusher. She watched in a mirror as a small patch of her baby's thick hair appeared and receded, appeared and receded, making gentle progress with each surge.

Four hours and 50 minutes into active labor, Arish and Emma welcomed their beautiful son. He was immediately presented to their guru's image and then lovingly examined from head to toe. A perfect little boy, complete with his mother's gorgeous hair and a dimple on his cheek.

As I left the hospital I felt a tide of gratitude sweep through me, as strong as any of Emma's surges, grateful to be part of this wonderful cycle of Life.

When I got home my husband asked how the birth had been. I replied, "I am Happy!" swept my hands downwards and laughed out loud. He looked at me sideways.

I have stayed in touch with Emma and Arish and look forward to watching the Happiest Baby on the Block grow up.

♀ The Doula High

by Nicola Wolters

It's 4:49 p.m. I'm on a birth doula high
I've got U2 on the radio playing "Beautiful Day"
It always is when I'm on my way to a birth
I'm more alive than ever at these times

Early-morning damp humidity of summer
Ice-cracking cold winter night
Each season special in its own way
Singing a greeting to the new baby

I'll be gone from home for so long
I left them with careful reassurances
Quick hugs, fleeting kisses to my 3 babies
Eye-contact with my husband – "you won't be long, will you?"

Mum's in active labor
"It's been like this for a whole day," she says
Maybe more…
It's been like this for two days now
Feels like forever and never

I hum to myself and to the almost-mother
"What is that you're humming?"
Beautiful Day, I carry it with me
"It is, isn't it?" she murmurs

Family flows in and out of her home with her contractions
They bring the day with them
Depart with it in their voices and hands
Holding her with them in love and anticipation

All this time I notice the laughter between mum and dad
Even when she is contraction-serious
She holds onto it through the hardest times
It's the world her baby already knows

A culmination of events strung together like beads
Each one defining a moment no less important than the other
A triumph of nature, miracles, chance
She is birthed into a circle of joy

Like a new little pebble she sends out ripples
Wonderful body-zinging electric currents of joy
Coursing through the lives of all her family
And her doula, always the doula

It's 1:18 a.m. I'm on a worn out, doula-ed-out high
I've got U2 on the radio playing "Beautiful Day"
It always is when I've just attended a birth
I'm more alive than ever at these times

A Heartbeat Away

by Raissa Chernushenko

♀

THIS TIME IT WAS DEFINITELY GOING to be a girl. Not because any ultrasound technician had given it away, not because I was determined by 90% of unsolicited opinions to be "carrying high," but simply because my father had said so.

You see, a curious family pattern had emerged over three generations, beginning with his own mother, who had birthed two children, a boy and then a girl. Each of them would grow up to have a girl first, then a boy, and now our generation had kept the alternating pattern going as my brother had completed his set of two – this time reverting back to the boy first. Five years earlier, I might have broken with tradition; however, my first pregnancy, a girl, sadly miscarried at 17 weeks gestation.

I then had my beautiful, bouncing boy, delivered almost two years later, after an exhausting 60 hours of stop and start labor. Originally intended as a home waterbirth, my water had broken five days after my due date and immediately after a hailstorm scare on the highway – eliminating any possible use of the rental birthing pool – with my labor concluding in the hospital aided by oxytocin. In fact, little by little, my entire birth-plan went down the drain.

My husband had been so sleep deprived from being my main support that he had not only brought the indoor carrier instead of the car seat to the hospital, but had briefly nodded off at the wheel on the way home to exchange it. So this time in addition to the care of a midwifery team we had vetoed the birthing pool but opted for the extra support of a doula assisted home birth.

Of course, with a toddler in tow, this pregnancy had not provided quite as much opportunity for practicing yoga, taking long contemplative baths, and fantasizing about whose eyes baby might have and whose wacky hammer-toes. I was more concerned with being reassured that I would be up to the task of enduring another marathon labor should that eventuality occur. The reality was that I would be celebrating my fortieth birthday three weeks before baby was due.

Not only was this my first doula, but I was to be her first official birth. She was very keen to get a sense of what kind of relaxation images and affirmations would be most helpful to me during labor, and I was impressed with her calm and humor. I took some of her suggestions and found some time to get out the pastel crayons and engage with a little of my own creativity, producing a rainbow-colored abstract drawing of a baby's head crowning.

As planned, a few days before my due date of November 11th or 12th, my mother came to visit, with the intention of helping look after my son during labor. By this time, my sacroiliac joint was giving me no end of grief, and I found it necessary to stop and stretch every ten meters. Long walks were out of the question, so I looked for other ways to distract myself, preferably not involving a dustcloth. A Christmas Craft Open House just down the street filled the bill nicely, but then Saturday evening came. How long would it be before we would get a couple's date again, we asked ourselves?

"But it's so close to the due date, maybe I'd better just stay home and rest," I said.

"We could go to a movie," my husband suggested. "*Serendipity* is playing."

"Oh don't worry about the baby coming," my mother reassured me. "She won't be here until the 12th. Haven't you noticed?

Everyone in your family has a birthday on an even numbered date, and everyone in your brother's family has an odd numbered date."

I did so want to believe her, not wishing a Remembrance Day birthday on my little one.

"Okay, *Serendipity* it is." I agreed, and waddled off to get my coat.

The fabulous thing about those last days of pregnancy is that you know you can allow yourself pretty well anything, diet-wise, especially at the movie refreshment stand. So we hunkered down to an unusually large supply of buttered popcorn and a mammoth root beer. About half an hour into the movie I noticed either a stomach cramp or a particularly intense Braxton Hicks contraction, but I'd been getting those several times a day for weeks. Caught up in the throes of a romantic movie, it wasn't until the end that I recalled having had several more and closer together. But from that point until bedtime they appeared to stop, and I truly thought nothing more about them.

At three o'clock the next morning – November 11th in fact – I sat upright and suddenly announced to my husband that I was pretty certain I was suddenly getting labor pains no more than five minutes apart and maybe – just maybe – he'd better call the doula. After all, she lived a considerable distance away. By the time he got off the phone, it was every three minutes and speeding along at a disconcerting pace. In fact, every time I stood or sat upright I was sent right into another contraction.

I groped my way down to my little "birthing suite" – the comfy nest I'd prepared in the basement where I practice shiatsu therapy – with a well protected futon and my birthing ball. I double checked all my supplies along with music choices and waited for someone to join me. At first, I felt a little irritated that for some time no one was there to keep me company or even ask what I might need. But soon I was swept into an internal orchestra of thoughts and feelings and waves of energy that appeared to be conducted by none other than my own voice. That low moaning, guttural animal sound I remember using to keep my lips relaxed during my first labor was back. The "Ohm" that is claimed to be the original sound of creation.

The baby is naturally doing what it should.

My uterus is contracting itself.

I welcome the pain.

I am relaxing into it, without tension, without sudden movement.

You are bringing my baby.

You are a good pain.

I had previously taken the trouble to type up these words in large bold print and post them on the wall.

But now my eyes were closed as I drifted in a world of my own, a whirl of both blackness and possibility, riding the tide of energy created by the excitement of knowing, of remembering that a baby would be a result of all this work. That this "being" was finding her way through the dark along the very same path that I was taking – just from the opposite end. It was so much easier to hold on to this image of working together, now that I had survived a previous birth.

Quite unexpectedly, my entire team of midwives had arrived before the doula appeared – team being the operative word. I had been previously told that not only two senior midwives, but two junior midwives in training would be present at the birth, and thought it sounded rather crowded. Suddenly it didn't seem to matter. I was so completely focused on my task I barely noticed the full house awaiting this mysterious little expected guest.

My poor husband had gone from being "primary support" in the birth of his baby to a mere bystander and door greeter. I floated and rocked – my inner world twirling like a gyroscope – both aware and somehow oblivious to the light hearted chatter and buzz of preparation around me. Time had collapsed and I seemed to exist on a plane that held all of the images of both of my previous labors in tandem with this snowballing, rocketing, free-fall joy ride. Only, this time, the fear was gone. I was flying, and flying alone.

Whether I took comfort in and found strength from the presence and wisdom of five other mothers, as well as my own mother, upstairs feeding breakfast to my son, or whether I had found the birthing zone on my own I can't quite recall, but what was actually 7 hours still to this day seems as though it were 7 minutes. I was not asked to do anything differently from what I was already innately doing. I chose when to stand and when to rest from my labor of love. I hung onto my doula for a few contractions, I asked what my son was eating, and smiled when I heard he was being treated to croissants for the very first time.

Suddenly transition began and I was gently encouraged to open my eyes. Had I really been in the dark for so long?

"Find a new outside focus," said the senior midwife. What better choice than my own vivid oil pastel drawing of "Crowning Glory" I had pinned to the wall just days before!

"Perfect." She said, as I gave up complete control.

Leaning against the very same wall was a small collection of hand drums I had collected, and the same senior midwife, being a drumming enthusiast herself, asked if I might like to have her play a heartbeat rhythm at this time. How perfect was that? My wee baby dancing her way down the final passage to the sound of the heartbeat of Mother Earth! I could not have thought of a more grounding and satisfying way to play out the last stage of birth.

So there I was, on the birthing stool, feeling as though I could have done this all alone, and yet cushioned by the encouraging energy of all present as I pushed until she was just a heartbeat away.

"Reach down and feel for baby's head now," I was told. I could actually be the first to touch her? To bring my baby out of her home and into mine with my very own hands?

So I did.

She was a girl after all, born into this world at 10 a.m. on November 11th, the day of all days to remember. When I called my father to tell him she was born, we still needed a middle name. He he jokingly said, "How about Poppy?"

We chose to call our little dancer Arianna Grace.

The Meaning of Water

by Jennifer Repec

MY BIRTH STORY BEGINS WITH death. After my sister's suicide by drowning, I started on the journey to slowly reclaim the beauty water had held for me before: a positive, healing, life-giving, and cleansing force. An avid swimmer and scuba diver, I found myself unable to dissociate her death from these sources of joy in my life. Then what seemed the ultimate way to mend my relationship with water and perhaps even my sister presented itself: actually giving birth to my first child in water.

The significance was lost on everyone else, and for that I was glad. When I realized this was the way I wanted to give birth, I didn't need the extra pressure of any ulterior issues. It was difficult enough to convince my partner and family that this was not only a safe method, but better for mother and child. The thought of a clinical, bright, impersonal hospital repelled me. My baby would be born in the warmth and security of our home.

How could I have my baby at home without the medical intervention that I dreaded? Wasn't someone going to prevent me? I had heard my mother's cautionary and dramatic story literally all my life, as she loved to recount her delivery of my sister in 1963 as a sort of David-and-Goliath triumph.

My mother had dared to fight with her obstetrician. At age 37, she was labeled an "elderly primigravida" (which struck her so funny she never forgot it). During contractions while strapped to a gurney, she resisted every time her obstetrician thrust a pen and release form in her face. He had suddenly decided after nine months of examinations that her pelvis was now too small and she would require a Caesarean. However, an x-ray showed that her pelvis was more than adequate and she was allowed to give birth.

At 43 years old and pregnant with my first child, I too had seen enough of hospitals to want to avoid them and try a natural birth. I did not want multiple ultrasounds; I certainly did not want invasive genetic testing. I had heard my mother's tirades and laments about her birth experiences all my life. Now who would help me shape my own experience?

I began with very good midwives, who had started their practice in other countries, places where midwifery was integrated into the healthcare system. Their perspectives gave me confidence in my decision and my body. And yet death continued to cast its shadow. During my third appointment at the midwife clinic, a routine check-up, a phone call came through from reception. Another pregnant woman was on the line for my midwife. "Can I take this call? It's urgent," she added. "Sure!" I chirped, trying to be agreeable while secretly wanting to get the appointment over with as quickly as possible.

"Oh. I'm so sorry," she began. "And the follow up tests? Yes. No. You have to wait until 20 weeks for burial. Before 20 twenty weeks it's considered a fetus. After 20. Yes. Well you can schedule that now..." I realized with growing horror that I was listening to a woman reporting the bad results of genetic testing, with the prospect of delaying termination for the fetus to develop into what a cemetery considered a baby old enough for burial!

And here I was concerned about the slight greenish tinge on my glucose test strip. I was humbled.

'It's okay," my midwife said after she got off the phone with the woman and heard my concern, "she has other children." Wow. That, I realized, was her reality as a seasoned midwife.

I was very fortunate. A woman I knew, pregnant at the same time as me, had miscarried at three months. This had spooked me, but also given me an added appreciation of what was happening with my own body. As I listened again to my mother's stories of regret, having no images of her own beautiful pregnant self, I made the decision to have maternity photos taken. As I met with photographers, one woman warned me her portfolio included babies born with terminal illness, done for no fee. Bereavement photography! I had never heard of such a thing, but it touched me so much I ended up working with her due in part to her obvious integrity. Death seemed inclined to wend its way through my birth experience.

Nine months. I had gotten this far. I had rented a birthing pool. It sat invitingly downstairs. Despite the qualms and outright skepticism of most family and friends, I was having my baby at home. Now I needed an ally, but it couldn't be someone I knew well. Anyone close would make me too conscious about my behavior during labor. I would be busy trying to seem okay so that they not worry about me, instead of letting myself go, freely, however the process unfolded. And I wanted a woman with such experience, confidence, and strength of character, that she could quell anyone's doubts and squash all the naysayers.

I needed a doula. I began my search carefully, allowing plenty of time. I met with doulas whose faces lit up when I mentioned my hope of a water birth. "Oh, I've always wanted to attend a water birth!" they all said. Uh oh, I thought. I did want to help these women learn, but I needed someone who was familiar with the process and could help me. And as an older woman, I also knew I would feel most comfortable with someone mature.

Six weeks passed. Holiday season was approaching, and it became difficult to set up appointments. I even tried meeting with multiple doulas in a pre-arranged group, and quickly realized these women were also looking for experience, and so young ... one woman had never attended a birth before! I was becoming frustrated. Perhaps I could manage without a doula.

I found her at the eleventh hour. I had a lead. Her biography was brief but to the point. She had assisted at more than 300 births. She came across as no-nonsense, but also kind and strong. By an amazing stroke of luck, she was available. I found a candid video of her online. She showed delight and a sense of fun. "That's her – my doula" I announced to my baby.

We met just two weeks before my due date! She was everything I had hoped for.

Our interview was in my home. I felt at ease with her right away. She was mature, with a wonderfully calm nature. But she was tough, too. An experienced doula, she wanted to know if I had known loss, and asked me frankly if I was prepared should things not go as I imagined for the birth. I liked that. She urged me to write out my birth plan, and also to know I must be prepared for all eventualities.

The first cramps came not two days after my official due date. As I woke feeling that familiar dull ache I used to experience during my menstrual cycle, I checked the time – 3:30 a.m. "I'm having cramps," I told my partner, and summarily fell into a deep sleep. Unbeknown to me, I had said the most alarming thing in the world! He woke up electrified and stayed wide awake until I got up again at 7:30 a.m.

"Are you ready to have a baby today?" I said as I hugged my partner after he came up the staircase. The look on his face – well, I thought to myself, this is why I have a doula.

"Don't you think you should call someone?" my partner asked. "Not yet." I reminded him that the midwives don't really want to know until the contractions begin. But my doula – this was her purpose. She had stressed that I call her anytime, for any reason. I could contact her without feeling I was being an alarmist. And so began our wonderful and reassuring communication, with emails and phone calls exchanged throughout the day.

By late that evening, after a lovely Thai curry supper, contractions had gotten more frequent. I phoned my doula and told her I needed her. She could be over to our house in 45 minutes. "I know

I'm having a baby, because my partner's vacuuming!" I laughed. "Take a picture," she advised. And I did. It's still one of my favorites.

I was beginning to get anxious. I sounded too calm on the telephone. I had waited too long. The doula would drive around for hours, lost in the icy, winding streets leading to the house. I distracted myself by doing a check of the birth supplies, making sure everything was really ready.

A ringing interrupted my first moment of doubt. "I'm almost there. Do you need anything before I arrive?" said the doula. Only 20 minutes! She had made record time. "No! See you soon!" I smiled with relief.

After she got to the house, my doula sat with us in the living room where I was shifting myself around, trying to find a way to ease the dull ache. "Try the floor," she suggested. "Okay." I laughed. "And it's so clean!" Lying there, I felt myself slowly losing focus on what was happening around me and turning my focus inward.

The women's singles match of the Australian Tennis Open was on TV. The effort of the serves, the grunts and cries, so primal, resonated with me.

"So when does real labor begin?" I asked drowsily. "You're *in* labor," she smiled, shaking her head slightly. "You're already there. I can tell you're somewhere else. You're doing everything you need to be doing." Her words washed over me, so calming and reassuring. "You want to think about calling the midwife now." That snapped me out of my state of calm. "Do I have to?" I thought to myself, and then said it out loud. Reluctantly, I went ahead and paged. No response in the ten minutes allotted. I called again, leaving another message. Finally the phone rang.

"How far apart?" It was the assistant midwife, referring to the frequency of my contractions. "Really?" More questions, and she talked about how her son had said, "You'd better go to bed mom – I bet there's going to be a birth." I realized she was listening to my voice as we spoke, gauging my progress. I knew I sounded too calm. I had an inspiration. "My DOULA says you should come," I emphasized, hoping that would convince her. "Oh, the doula's there? Okay." What a relief! And what a boon having a doula was turning out to be!

Off the phone and having put the wheels in motion, I wanted nothing more than to strip and immerse myself in the warm, soothing water. "Do you really want to get in?" my doula asked. "Yes! But she told me not to." I recounted how the midwife's assistant had asked me to wait until after they arrived before getting in the pool. "Go on, get in," my doula urged me.

The glee I felt! I never would have had the courage to do it without her endorsement. The pleasure of sinking into that water! All the ache of contractions melted away. How wonderful to float – the sheer novelty of being weightless and bobbing around made me giddy. I was doing it! I was really having our baby at home.

What luxury! And how surreal. When else in my life would I be in my house, relaxing in a warm pool, watching one of my favorite movies? I had chosen a classic to have on while I labored: *The Thirty-Nine Steps*, an old, familiar film to which I knew all the dialog by heart. Friends had advised me to watch a comedy to pass the time during labor, but this had that old-style dry wit and suspense, too. Curiously, I was to begin hard labor only after the movie finished.

These things were a comfort to me, but they proved even better for my partner as much-needed distractions. He got the movie going and spent the evening boiling pots of water to keep the pool warm when our water tank proved to be heating too slowly (something the pool rental company had alerted us about ahead of time, thankfully!) He had not wanted the water birth, but knew how important it was to me. In the end, he himself tended to the pool and made sure it was perfect for me.

The doula's role quickly shaped itself. I knew she was there to care for me; I just wasn't sure how this would manifest itself. After the midwife and student midwife arrived, my baby's vital signs needed to be checked frequently. I was having to lift myself out of the warm comfort of the water each time. It was so disruptive I must have said out loud, "I wish I could just stay in." Suddenly my doula was convincing the midwives that they could safely immerse the waterproof fetal heart rate monitor; she promised it would be fine. What a relief! My advocate! And they let me stay in my pool.

With the middle of the night approaching and my body undulating with heavier contractions, I began vocalizing. As the women did with each serve at the Australian Open, I let out a mighty yell with each effort. It was perfect, like white noise; I could block out any chatter around me and concentrate on myself.

Although the midwife made comments about the neighbors hearing the noise, my doula was right there with her support. "You're doing a great job!" she encouraged me. "Those are good sounds." Meanwhile she had been carefully filming and taking photos as I had asked her to do, as well as continually checking in to see if I needed anything.

Things progressed quickly. As the hush of deep night took hold, there was real quiet as my contractions got much stronger with long, peaceful breaks. It was almost reverential, and made me really aware that something absolutely miraculous was happening: birth.

By a huge effort I spoke, carefully forming my words to be as succinct as possible: "I would assume that these longer pauses between contractions means the baby will be coming soon," I told, rather than asked the four who were witnessing the birth. A rustle and the women circled in close. "Oh yes" said my midwife, as I saw eager faces, getting ready.

A push and the head! My first moment of feeling outside my body again, a pain that shook me from my reverie. I urged my partner to touch the amazingly pliant, round firmness of our baby's head. "Dark hair," murmured the midwife. I smiled. Good. Just like all the babies in our family.

Three more minutes and the baby was out in one mighty push! And into the water and outstretched hands. A boy!

"A boy," laughed my partner and I together. We had really had no idea at all. I was fascinated by the wonder on his stunned face, this man who was unflappable.

This baby on my chest was so like my sister! It must be wishful thinking. I held him and gazed into his face. Yes, so much like her.

I needed to tell my mother that everything was okay. Even at

3:30 in the morning, I felt she would be awake, waiting for the news. And she was. For the first time I wept. Relating how well everything went and telling her about her grandson made me realize in a rush of emotion all that had just taken place.

My birth story will always be a part of me, something I feel privileged to have shared with those who were there with me and now can relate to others. How gratifying to be told by each woman who helped me that it was an honor to attend my labor.

I know that something more than luck brought us all together and made everything go smoothly. I did achieve the healing I sought, with the blessing of a healthy baby born the way I had imagined. The true fulfillment of my dream of a perfect birth.

Echo

by Lisa Doran

SHE IS NAKED AND PANTING AND sweating. Working so very hard. Another contraction begins. Her eyes snap open.

"Lisa!" she pants. "I can't do this."

"Melissa," I say. "Look at me."

She looks at me as her contraction peaks, and I can see that she is struggling, I can see that she is suffering, I can sense that she is reaching what she perceives is her limit.

"You can do this," I say, and I open myself up completely to her in that moment and I let her see that I have been where she is at this moment and I let her see that I understand her struggle and her suffering. That she is safe, that I am here for her and that she is strong. I also let her see that if she is willing to dig even deeper that her "self" is capable of enduring this.

Her contraction subsides.

She laughs.

"You have done this before," she says. Meaning that I have lived the moment she is living now, finding my limit – learning to reach past it and transform my pain and fear and exhaustion into motivation and ecstasy. Yes. I have been there. Joy, pain, ecstasy, transformation.

"Here comes the next one." Her tone of voice shows that what she means is, "I am ready."

> I can't do this.
> It's too hard.
> This is more work than I thought it would be.
> It hurts. I feel uncomfortably out of control.
> I am hot. It's too hard.
> I look at Tim.
> "I can't do this," I plead.
> And he simply takes me in his arms and runs his fingers lovingly through my hair and he whispers: "You can do this."
> We cling together and sway together. Connected in this moment, bound together absolutely in the experience of the birth of our second child.
> And I remember to breathe.
> It is that simple.
> What he conveys in his perfect statement and through his touch is unconditionally this: I trust you, I love you, I am here for you. You are strong.
> I breathe again. Here comes the next one. I am ready.

She is slow-dancing with her midwife to the rhythm of contractions. Hands on hips her midwife reminds her how to sway and move her baby down. I squat in the corner in the dark and watch this ancient and familiar dance. It is in my bones too. This knowing. They are dancing, forehead to forehead. Women gathering. We hold the space. Murmer murmer. Gentle secret. Midwife holds her, midwife guides her. Mama leads.

> Men.
> Men who soften as they tend to their wives or simply crack wide open as they hold their blood and vernix covered daughters in their big hands.

Men who cry at birth.

Strong men who gentle their birthing women like I've seen a scared horse gentled; softly, softly in wonder of this powerful creature. Open hearted and connected.

Courageous men who have reached the point where they know and accept that they cannot fix the situation or make it better or rescue their beloved. This journey is hers and they will keep her safe and protect the space and will calm and support her because they know instinctively that this is the only way to get through. This is hers alone. Surrender and acceptance is difficult for most men but sometimes surrender is the only way through.

They are pounding on the bathroom door.

"Do you want me to call 911?"

I grunt "No." I know the midwives are on their way. We are OKAY.

"What is going on in there?"

"Baby," I gasp as the first spontaneous push causes my entire body to bear down.

I feel the burn of my baby crowning as I am standing leaning against the bathroom sink. I reach down and feel his head between my legs. All I can think of is to hold his head. My legs won't hold me anymore, so I squat down onto the toilet – the only close-by support as another powerful contraction moves through me. I feel him wet and wiggle out. I hear him splash into the toilet.

Now silent and pure calm instinct takes over. Things become surreal. Somehow I know exactly what to do. I don't hear my husband at the door. In fact, I don't hear anything. I lift my baby to my chest. He is grey and soft. I suck the mucous from his mouth and nose. I turn him over and rub his back. I sing gently, "hello baby hello baby," and suddenly he is pink and flexing his arms and legs and crying. I am dripping blood and fluid and shaking, holding my pink and squalling newborn whose cord and placenta are still inside of me. Adrenaline surges and I am powerful. I feel like an amazon goddess warrior!

My midwife arrives dashing up the stairs to an excited welcome from my 3 year old. We HAD a baby he proclaims. I am tucked into bed and I gaze blissfully at my third son. I am in love as the world rushes and frets around me. We are OKAY. Of course.

We are pushing. Eyes screwed tight, lips pursed more tightly. Tension in every muscle. Resisting.

I push too, I almost can't help it, mirroring her effort – and then I feel the tension in my body, my shoulders, my yoni. I remember my Ina May and I know what is missing. There is power here but birth should also be beautiful Ina May says, or there is something that needs correcting.

"Sarah," I whisper, "Sarah, look at me."

Because when you are pushing with this wild feeling in your breast sometimes watching is easier than words.

She opens her eyes and I grin at her. Her eyes communicate momentary incomprehension at this doula-friend who is nose to nose and grinning. And then it dawns on her and I see she understands. She remembers Ina May too – we have talked about it together, heads bent over our lattes one cold winter afternoon 4 months ago. Talked about the beauty in birth.

She closes her eyes and collects herself and when she opens her eyes she smiles. She smiles with all of herself – thoughts, eyes and heart. She is angelic, radiant, beautiful. There it is. All is good.

I sigh.

The room shifts, brightens somehow.

Her body softens and relaxes.

Little boy crowns.

All is good.

♀ Left Brain / Right Brain

by Shawn Gallagher

*"Optimum labor requires [women] to enter into a trance state –
not a logical, thinking state"* – Ina May Gaskin

A pregnant mum who wants to relax
a hypnotist guiding the process...
and everything else in between

> *just get comfortable*
> *and as you do...*
> *take a long ... slow ... deep breath*
> *down into your toes*
> *filling all the cells of your body with calm...*
> *and peace...*
> *and relaxation*

THIS IS NUTS – I CAN'T RELAX.
THE SECOND I TRY, ALL THE CLOWNS PILE OUT OF THE TINY
CAR.
REMEMBER ME – THIS NEEDS TO BE DONE – OVER HERE,
OVER HERE – LOOKIT MEEEE!
CLOWN THOUGHTS.

> *the music in the background calming you ... so peaceful...*

AAARRRGH

> *just letting go...*
> *relaxing into the surface beneath you...*
> *every breath ... every word takes you deeper and deeper...*

STOP THINKING – STOP THINKING – STOP THINKING.
EVERYTHING'S ITCHY. CAN'T GET COMFORTABLE.
WAIT A MINUTE, WHAT WAS THAT?
AN EASIER BIRTH?
HUH. THAT'LL BE THE DAY.

...deeper and deeper into relaxation...
your subconscious mind is open and receptive to positive...
helpful... and beneficial suggestions
of a safe and natural birth...
every uterine surge creates more natural anaesthetic...
every rest period takes you deeper and deeper into calm...
and comfort...

I *WOULD* LIKE AN EASIER BIRTH – THAT WOULD BE LOVELY.
IF –
IF IT WERE DOABLE ... LOOK, IT'S A NICE IDEA, BUT REALLY!
WHAT'S THAT THING THEY SAY IN THE BIBLE?
IT'S WHY THEY CALL IT LABOR.
THAT TOP OBSTETRICIAN. WHAT DID HE SAY IN THE MAGAZINE?
THE MAN'S GOT TO BE A SAINT TO HAVE TO DEAL WITH
THOSE HOMEBIRTH NUTS.
I WOULD NEVER DO ANYTHING TO JEOPARDIZE MY BABY'S
SAFETY.

[factoid: *Macleans* used to be called "The Busy Man's Magazine."
Controversy for the sake of publicity?
After all, it's not a science magazine.
They can write what they want.
I guess anything to boost sales – even scaring pregnant women
with birth gone wrong stories.]

and as you relax, your baby relaxes...
and receives the best
of your body's natural...
and safe...

ENDORPHINS … AND OXYTOCIN…
GOOD FOR YOU … GOOD FOR YOUR BABY…
RELAXING AND BEING CALMER
REDUCES THE FIGHT-FLIGHT-FREEZE CHEMICALS IN ME
THAT'S GOT BE GOOD FOR MY BABY, DOESN'T IT?

… and as you get to your due date…

MY WHAT? DUE DATE?
SO MUCH LEFT TO DO!!
TIME SLIPPING AWAY…
GOTTA RELAX.
RELAX. BREATHE. BREATHE. RELAX.

after 37 completed weeks…
to a week or so past your due date…
is Term…

CALL THE STORE. THAT SPECIAL ORDER NEEDS TO GO IN THIS
WEEK.
AND PUT A FIRE UNDER SOMEBODY'S TAIL … S-O-M-E-B-O-D-Y
HAS TO PAINT BABY'S ROOM. NOW. NO MORE EXCUSES.
I'M NOT READY, I'M NOT READY, I'M NOT READY … OMG I'M
SO NOT READY. :(

Your subconscious mind keeps everything closed and tight until
term
Your baby safely stays inside until term
and tell your subconscious mind to create natural anaesthetic
and make sure baby is born safely…
at term…
in the setting of your choice…

HOW DO WOMEN DO THIS?
I'M A BASKET CASE.
…BASKET CASE … BASKET CASE … BASKET…

...BABY BASKET ... HA HA ... BABY SAFELY INSIDE ...
HAHAHA...
WAIT A MINUTE! WHO AM I KIDDING?
I CAN'T DO THIS.
NATURAL BIRTH? THEY'VE GOT TO BE NUTS.
...NUTS ... I'M HUNGRY ... SOME IN MY PURSE?... ALWAYS SO
HUNGRY...
IT'S NOT POSSIBLE. STUPID NATURAL BIRTH CRAZIES.
THANK GOD FOR EPIDURALS.
GOTTA PEE.
EVERYONE SAYS ... *EVERYONE SAYS* ... DON'T LEAVE HOME
WITHOUT IT.
BLESSED EPIDURALS. :)
I'VE BEEN SO GOOD THIS PREGNANCY ... NOT EVEN ONE
ACETAMINOPHEN...
...IT WILL BE SO NICE... TO GO NUMB...
TO BE COMPLETELY COMFORTABLE FOR A CHANGE...
THEY SAY YOU CAN SLEEP, IT'S THAT COMFORTABLE.
AND SAFE, THEY SAY. THE BEST OF MODERN-DAY MEDICINE.
CADILLAC, THEY SAY.
SURE, "NATURAL" ... I'M JUST SAYING...

...deeper and deeper ... imagine you are at term...
in the setting of your choice...
everybody there and ready...
everything opens easily...
...comfortably ... your body's natural anaesthetic...
good for you ... good for your baby...
relaxing deeper and deeper to your partner's touch...
you are safe...
you are loved...
all is well...

MAYBE..
WHAT IF THIS IS POSSIBLE?
WHAT IF MY BODY CAN DO THIS?

ALL I NEED TO DO IS RELAX … ALLOW IT TO HAPPEN.
NOT FIGHT IT.
I CAN DO "CALM" … I'M OKAY WITH THAT…
NOT SURE ABOUT THE ORGASMIC THOUGH…
THAT WOULD BE WEIRD…

[Thousands of years of hypnotic commands to women to suffer.
There is so much dehypnotizing to do.
Joyful birth sometimes feels like creating a ladder to the moon.
The endless generations of dna programming
to unwind and reprogramme.
And then pregnant women wrap themselves in their fears
and argue for their limitations.

I wonder – is there anything I have missed?
Is every part of her subconscious okay with natural and normal
birth?

So many years of our culture not understanding birth.
Of men trying to improve on nature.
Of women begging to be saved from their bodies.
Of medicine misunderstanding the needs of birthing women
a medical hierarchal structure of those who have power
and those who do not.
And women not speaking up for what they need.]

imagine your baby in your arms…
you did it … your beautiful baby … safely
in your arms…
you and your partner and your baby
you are all safe…
you are all loved…
all is well…

[I need to be positive for her.
She needs confidence in herself.

Be supportive, be caring.
Nurture her and her baby will be nurtured.]

jUST RELAXING ... GOODNESS THIS FEELS NICE...
I'M OKAY, MY BABY IS OKAY...
CLOWNS ... IN BASKETS ... BABIES ... IN BASSINETS ... LOL...
WE ARE SAFE ... WE ARE LOVED...
IT WILL BE OKAY...
I CAN DO THIS ... BABY LOVES ME ... PARTNER LOVES ME ...
WE ARE A FAMILY...
A TEAM ... DOING THIS TOGETHER...

> *and as you emerge...*
> *back to full awareness...*
> *keeping the best of the positive suggestions...*
> *releasing what no longer serves you...*
> *you may feel stronger...*
> *more confident...*
> *more capable...*

WE ARE ALL SAFE...
WE ARE ALL LOVED...
ALL IS WELL...
I CAN DO THIS...

> *FIVE ... coming out*

I AM DOING THIS...

> *FOUR ... back to full alertness...*

ONCE I PUT MY MIND TO IT, I CAN RELAX, I CAN

> *THREE ... wiggle your fingers ... wiggle your toes...*

NO ... NO ... NO ... I WANT TO STAY HERE ... IT FEELS SO
GOOD...

TWO ... fully alert ... give a stretch ... coming back ... take a deep
breath...

IF MY HYPNOTIST/DOULA THINKS I CAN DO THIS, PERHAPS I
CAN...

and ONE ... back to full awareness...fully alert ... opening your
eyes...
Back in the room.
Feeling wonderful.

WELL THAT WAS NICE.
I FEEL RELAXED.

Wonderful! You seem to relax well once you settle in.
I think you are very capable of birthing this baby.
Remember, we all have this ability.

[She relaxes nicely.
I hope this helps.
I really hope she has a lovely birth.
It's a fine line – optimism and hope ... balanced with realism.
Everyone is different – different needs, different strengths.
One day ... some day...
everyone will have a safe and natural and comfortable birth.
"We women are not machines," says Ina May Gaskin.
Women need warmth, and privacy, and to feel safe and respected
and loved.]

Our bodies naturally create endorphins for comfort.
And oxytocin for birth and breastfeeding.
Did you know that oxytocin is called the Love Hormone?

REALLY?

It's part of bonding
and your body makes it naturally
for you and your baby
plus it is good for your baby.
The biggest pharmacy on the planet is the one between your ears.

I HAD NO IDEA.

More and more women are reporting these amazing births.
It's probably been going on for a very long time.
It's just nobody has been talking about it.

THAT'S INTERESTING.

What does a joyful birth mean to you?

WELL…

A Lesson in Birth

by Kirsten Perley

AS I SIT DOWN TO WRITE, I WONDER if my voice, the voice of a labor and delivery registered nurse, is a voice that should be heard in this forum. I question my contribution knowing that my lens may have a different color and my words a slightly different dialect among the other voices of birth. I ask you to follow along in my journey with me as I tell the story of how I figured out what it truly meant to be with a woman in labor.

It had been a slow start to the shift, not a usual day on my unit that was usually busting at the seams with patients. I returned from my morning break and received my assignment from my charge nurse: a primip with pre-labor rupture of membranes 1 centimeters dilated and 50% effaced who was positive for GBS. I went to the triage room to get the report and then went up to the couple to introduce myself. I was met with a very tense looking husband who seemed like he might explode at any minute, and the patient herself had her head hung low almost in shame. My outstretched hand was met with air, neither the patient nor the husband reached out their hands to meet mine. This was not the usual response I had upon meeting a patient and their family for the first time. I am always acutely aware of context so I inquired if there was something wrong.

The husband spat at me that his wife had just been examined by a male physician and that was deeply offensive in his culture. "We go to a female obstetrician; why was she examined by a male?" I apologized for the circumstances, which did not help. They were aware that nothing could change the fact that there was no female OB on call that day. He looked at me with disgust. This cultural clash is something that occurred on occasion, and whenever it could be avoided, as nurses we did our best to respect the wishes of the patients. Today, however, was a holiday and the only OB on was a man. I asked a few questions and discovered that the patient spoke very little English; her husband was acting as a translator. I then explained we would now go to the birthing suite so that the patient and her family could settle in.

The patient was comfortable in terms of pain as she was only having some mild cramping. I showed her how to navigate walking and pushing the IV pole that was holding up the antibiotics. I then asked the husband if he would collect their belongings and follow us. He put his hand up in my face: "That's not my job–that is women's work." I could feel my temper rise with my eyebrows my jaw set as I wanted to say: "Well I'm an RN and that's not my job." I explained that he could move them in or not but I would not be moving them. Acid almost burned from his eyes as he opened the door of the triage room and yelled for his mother to come and collect their bags and coats. My feminist blood was boiling, I'm sure my mouth was agape all the while I'm thinking wow, ten more hours of this to go, this is going to be a great day.

We arrived at the birthing suite and I oriented them to all the usual things – how the recliner worked and where the call bell was. Then I explained the plan for pitocin induction and what that meant, and how it would use the same IV that the patient already had in her arm. "This is not how we do this in my country" was the response I received from the husband. I offered to have the doctor come and speak to them again and perhaps we could offer some different options. The husband merely glared back at me. I completed all the routine intake questions while monitoring the fetal heart rate. I then asked permission to start the pitocin. The patient looked to her husband to respond. His response was just as acerbic as his prior ones: "Whatever, do what you must." I started the pitocin and quickly left the room. Just nine and a half hours more....

I finished up the initial admission paper work and then went in for the half hour check. Nothing had changed yet as it so rarely does until about the 3 hour mark and then whammo! Insanely painful contractions that no one can deal with. I entered the room taking a deep breath trying not to add any fuel to the fire. It went on like this for about 2 hours, entering the room with a glaring husband and mother-in-law who would watch me with disapproval each time I increased the pitocin. Each time they would gesture at me and make comments in their language. I can't say for sure what they were saying but let's assume it wasn't anywhere near positive. The patient sat there with head held low and never looked at me nor responded when I asked how she was doing. It was lunch time now and I gladly headed for break.

When I returned from lunch, the patient was starting to get uncomfortable. I pulled up my chair and demonstrated different techniques for coping, limited as they are when you are on fetal monitor and have an IV. I offered to apply counter pressure to the patient's hips and sacrum. She accepted but she didn't like it. I showed her husband and encouraged him and his mother to try. No dice. I left the room to check another patient ... I had barely been out of the room 1 minute before the call bell went off. I went back in, explaining I would be back and that I was covering for another nurse. The husband stomped up to me and yelled in my face: "Do something for her!" My eyes were wide and I'd had enough. "Just what would you like me to do for her?" "Do something, make it better!" "Get the doctor!" he yelled emphatically, my wife is having the baby!" "No sir she is in labor, she probably has another 7 to 8 hours of this before she has the baby." I had to go and check another patient, I explained, and I would be back in 5 minutes. The bell was ringing before I could even get back. The impatience and fury was now even more frenetic. "Do something right now, I demand it!"

"Well I can't really do anything! Your wife is in labor and, this is what has to happen to have the baby."

"Well make it better!" he yelled. Well the only thing that will make it "better" in terms of pain is an epidural. I actually never offer an epidural; I talk about it when a woman initially comes in but I never offer one. I don't want to be the voice that tells a woman that she can't do it and undermine her confidence in her own body. This is one of those cases where I figured I would offer an epidural. The husband's response was "absolutely not, she is meant to suffer through this."

Oh great, here we go, this is my favorite scenario, a culture where the women have no say and the men decide all the details of their labors. I'm certain I was literally biting my tongue by this point, I responded by saying it wasn't his choice it was hers. Looking at the patient who seemed to understand more English than she could speak, I knew it really wasn't her choice. I was sickened by this husband; he seemed cruel and uncaring and I was frankly sick of how he was treating me. How dare he stand in front of me and speak to me this way. I felt anger on so many levels for his anti-woman behavior, however, I wasn't there to look after him. My responsibility was mom and babe.

I offered to examine the patient to see how far along she was as that could sometimes help guide a decision on pain management. I checked and she had done beautifully 4 centimeters and 100% effaced. I explained that she was doing great but that it would still most-likely be a number of hours to get to 10 centimeters and then another 1 to 2 hours of pushing. By now the patient was shrieking and trying to climb the bed with each contraction. The husband was yelling at me each time his wife shrieked and his mother would join in every once in a while just for good measure. The answer to pain meds was a definitive no! I sat in the room with them coaching on breathing. The patient would glare at me the whole time, and then shriek and then the husband would yell. I would gratefully leave every 30 minutes for the respite that checking on another patient afforded me. A quick bathroom break or a drink of water and several deep breaths and then I would enter the room again. The response was always the same, glaring, shrieking and yelling. Wow 3 more hours until the end of shift....

The tension in the room was palpable and I did my best not to betray the anger I was still holding toward the husband because he was still being inappropriate in terms of his comments towards me. After one really intense contraction where the shrieking and yelling had reached a deafening crescendo, I snapped. "Sir you need to stop – you're not actually allowed to speak to me like that. It's not helpful either." He sat in shocked silence. His wife was shrieking again, and I tried in vain to explain again that lower toned growls or moans would be more helpful in aiding dilation. The husband at this point was refusing to translate. Not to be out done, I decided to demonstrate it to the patient who nodded her head in acknowledgment. After a couple of contractions the patient started to push involuntarily. There were no other signs that she was fully dilated, such as more bloody show or that moment that a women suddenly heads into transition and you know she is almost ready without ever examining. I asked permission to examine her cervix and found her to be the same still at 4 centimeters. This news caused an uproar with all involved. The patient was back to shrieking, the husband back to yelling, and the mother-in-law was vociferously joining in. I sat beside the patient thinking, what can I do? They are not willing to work with me, she doesn't want me to rub her back, she doesn't want me to coach her breathing, she doesn't want an epidural. I have nothing else that I can do. I sat there at the bedside for about 5 minutes not looking at anyone, not engaging them in their yelling, not doing anything, not even charting. I had been doing a meditation class and I decided that meditation to just calm myself down at this point couldn't hurt. I closed my eyes, grounded myself, and breathed deeply into my abdomen. I filled my belly deeply with each breath and then visualized myself connected to the earth. Once I had reached that still point where I could feel there was space in my brain and peace in my heart, I asked for guidance. "What do you want me to do?" I asked the question silently. I was startled when I received a response, "Nothing, just bear witness." The words were not familiar to me, not words I would use. I continued to breathe as I opened my eyes and then realized my surroundings had changed. Everyone seemed calmer, the husband was no longer yelling but rather he was gently encouraging his wife, she was moaning in lowered guttural tones and her body was relaxing, she was no longer climbing up the bed. The mother-in-law smiled at me. I sat in my chair at the bedside doing and being nothing but calm, connected, and positive.

After an hour of doing and being nothing, breathing and bearing witness, the patient made that sound, the sound that tells you she's fully dilated. She started to push, everyone in the room was working together now, encouragement was everywhere. The pushing was not easy, it seemed a rather large baby was trying to present itself. The husband was mopping her brow and getting ice chips for her. He seemed excited and happy now. After 2 hours of hard pushing, the baby was starting to crown. I told them I would be calling the doctor. The mood started to change. "It will be a man?" he quietly asked. "Yes I believe it will be, I'm sorry about that." I genuinely felt how disappointed they all were, I was disappointed for them, knowing it would erase all that had been achieved. I put on the call bell and asked for help. The patient was working well with her contractions, she was in her zone allowing her body to open up and do what it needed to do. The door opened, I noticed I had been holding my breath. I was feeling their mounting tension over an unknown male entering their space. I looked up to see a nurse from the night shift and right behind her one of our female obstetricians. Sweet mercy it was shift change for both the nurses and the OB's. The patient was going to get her unmedicated birth and a female obstetrician to boot. A collective relief flooded over the patient and her family, and a few pushes later their very beautiful son was born. I stayed for the birth and to congratulate her on all her hard work. As I said goodbye to the family, the husband came and shook my hand and the mother-in-law gave me a huge smile. I left that birth permanently altered. I have been a participant in thousands of births, but this one taught me the most.

The old me would have allowed the power struggle to continue, and I would have let my anger and indignation rule my behavior with this family. At this birth, I learned that sometimes it was most important to do nothing but be present and in the moment. At this birth, a sense of non-judgement, unconditionally loving and grounded presence was what was needed to allow birth to occur. I walked away knowing that something really important had been achieved for both the patient and myself.

Summer Night

by Kendra Smith

♀

MY PASSION FOR BIRTH AND LABOR was preceded by my curiosity of death and dying. I suppose it is the significance of how one's soul enters and exits this life that intrigues me. I attended a conference for support workers on the subject of death and dying and I heard a phrase that has always stayed with me: "The best thing you can do is walk into that room like there is nothing wrong happening there." Ironically, it seems our society fears the process of both birth and death. These shifts of consciousness into or out of the physical body can be more comforting in the calming presence of a support person, and that's when the idea to become a birth doula hit me.

Birth is a sacred occasion in life and many cultures honor it as such. Women need support and encouragement on the journey of giving birth. They need someone to walk into the room, look them in the eye and let them know there is nothing wrong happening. To show them what they're going through is nothing short of a miracle, and they are strong enough.

As I rushed through the Emergency doors of the hospital that warm summer's night, I giggled at what I must look like to by-standers: a duffle bag full of ice packs, heat packs, massage rollers, peppermint essential oil for nausea, knee pads for kneeling, crocs on my feet for easy cleaning after the occasional splash of broken waters, and a big bouncy pink birthing ball under my arm.

I am greeted by the voice of a female security guard sitting behind a desk. "Excuse me can I help you?" she says with a confused expression on her face. "Hi I'm a doula, my client is in labor, and I'm heading up to the maternity floor." A pause.... "A dou-whata?" I wish a perfect definition quickly rolled off my tongue, but instead in the haste of getting upstairs to my client all I could manage was a swift "you know, like a birth coach." The security guard nodded hesitantly and insisted on accompanying me up to the maternity floor, explaining that it is a special floor that deserves extra safety and attention.

This was my first birth with nurses and an obstetrician rather than with midwives and I was nervous because of all the unnecessary medical intervention horror stories I had heard from friends. I slowly entered the dimly lit private whirlpool room where my client Margo lay naked against her husband Rob, submerged in warm soothing water, waging the battle of intense rushes. Margo was making high-pitched groans at the peak of each rush, and I quietly reminded her to focus on deep low sounding moans and keeping her mouth and lips loose. She took this direction and stated afterwards that she believes it really sped up the process of dilation.

The love and support between Margo and Rob at this pivotal time in their lives was incredible. Rob lost himself in the ebb and flow of Margo's labor rushes, becoming still and quiet during the rush and then whispering loving words of encouragement in her ear and brushing hair from her face during periods of relaxation. After an hour of this routine, Margo began falling asleep for one minute intervals in between rushes. I could see the tension and intensity of the rush slowly leave her body, her eyes would flutter closed and then her head would gently fall back onto her husband's chest behind her. It was female instinct at its best, conserving the body's energy and falling into complete relaxation in between rushes. I believe being in water really helps with this process.

Margo and Rob were coping beautifully, so much so that I mostly just sat with them holding space and occasionally offered words of encouragement. I began to question whether I was even necessary, when out of the blue Margo's head fell back against Rob's chest and she looked over at me with pleading eyes and said, "Thank you so much for being here with us." This simple statement at 6 centimeters dilated was enough to remind me why I love being a doula. My presence there was reassuring for her, and her gratitude for me is why I don't hesitate to get out of bed at 3:00 a.m. to rush to a birth.

Margo reached transition within a few hours of her first rush, which was surprising to me for two reasons: first, labor generally lasts longer for a first birth, and second, she was coping so well with each rush. If it wasn't for the frequency and timing of the rushes, I wouldn't have believed she was in transition. During a particularly intense rush, a nurse with lovely nurturing energy entered the room and explained that we needed to check dilation. When Margo refused to get out of the tub, the nurse chuckled and checked her while she was in the whirlpool. The nurse smiled. "Okay, the babies ready, we need to get you out of the tub." Margo was at 10 centimeters and ready to push after 3 hours of un-medicated labor! Margo did not want to get out of that tub – you should have seen the look on her face getting out of the tub and into the wheel chair. At one point, she shrieked, "The baby's going to fall out of me!" ...if only it was that easy.

This is by far my favorite part of the birthing process, the pushing stage. All of the excitement, fear, and hard work reaches its peak. Mothers usually say that this stage feels good (with the exception of the 'ring of fire') because it is productive and fruitful – they are so close to meeting their baby. Partners and doulas anxiously take their place beside mom to cheer her on, hold her hand, take pictures, and prepare to cut the umbilical cord.

Margo began pushing with every ounce of strength she had in her body. After every few pushes, she would look up at me as if to say, "Like this? Am I doing this right?" I squeezed her thigh and kept eye contact with an expression of unwavering confidence. At one point she moaned, "I can't do this," and I simply replied "You ARE doing it." The OB entered the scene at this point, and just as she had whipped her gloves on and began massaging the perineum around the babies crowning head, a voice came over the P.A system "Dr. Evans we need you in room 10," the nurse looked up at her and said "Go, it's a multip in room 10, you know how those babies just slide out, we've still got time here." And just like that Dr. Evans vanished from the room and the nurses took over.

Margo watched the OB leave and then looked at me as though she should stop pushing until Dr. Evans came back, but her body and this baby had other ideas. She could not and did not stop pushing. Margo kept saying "it feels so good to push." After 15 minutes, Dr. Evans raced back into the room, slapped on a fresh pair of gloves, and caught the silent baby. Everything happened so fast.

The moment Margo and Rob's beautiful baby girl began crying, Margo's head fell back against the pillow, eyes closed in exhausted relief, her baby girl placed on her chest. This is the moment during birth that gets me every time; I felt my eyes welling up as I watched magnificent love envelop this baby and her mother. It is the moment where Rob and Margo looked at their baby girl with such devotion, and realized nothing will ever compare to the love they feel for this child. They smiled and kissed each other – a brand new family. I smiled in disbelief that I was fortunate enough to be part of this monumental day in their lives. At this point, their baby girl had started up with a loud gurgly cry. Margo looked at Rob and said, "Goodbye sleep." They both laughed.

As I drove home from the hospital with the sun rising in my rear view mirror, the adrenalin began to wear off and the fatigue began to set in – a satisfied fatigue. I was content with life at that very moment. That is what attending births will do to you; it will help you breathe in and live in the present moment and help you remember that each life is a gift. More than anything I believe a good experience during labor helps remind women that they are capable of anything, that they are stronger and more powerful than they can even imagine. Although my game face during births is one of poise and reassurance, after every birth I am still constantly in awe of the innate strength and courage of women to birth their children. Witnessing a new life entering this world is moving beyond words. As a doula I am so honored to share in that miracle.

♀ Pulse

by Joanne Dahill

Dusk light
to
Moon light
to
Star light
to
Dawn light

to the pulse of the cosmos she dances.

She mews.
She moans.
She moves
to sensations
that for centuries
have called forth

The coming

The coming

The crowning

The birthing

The beating
of a heart newly-formed
now born
to be among us.

Authors Note: I wrote this poem on December 23, 2007. I was reflecting upon all the births that I had witnessed throughout the past year and wanted to send a note to the mothers to thank them for allowing me to be present at such an intimate, profound, and, in my mind, sacred time of life.

She Never Imagined

by Jody Cummins-Lambert

THE FIRST NOTEWORTHY CONTRACT-ion had hit her while she was standing in the waiting area of the midwife's office. She had just been introduced to a newly pregnant woman attending her first appointment, and while in the midst of initial "nice to meet you's" she had struggled to focus on the words coming out of the other woman's mouth, a slight ringing in her ears from the intensity of whatever had just happened in her body. She didn't realize that this was "it"!

There had been too many false starts in the days before, and so she figured this was just another annoying twinge, albeit a doozy. Her midwife, a divine earth mother type with silver hair and an ever glowing twinkle in her eyes, was slated to leave for London in two days and had called that afternoon with a cancellation in her schedule, asking her to come in to see where things were at. Now here she was standing in the waiting room trying to focus on the conversation without anyone noticing that anything was out of the ordinary. She walked upstairs with her mother and the midwife to an intimate clinic office where she lay down to have her cervix "stretched and swept," after which her midwife knowingly smiled and said, "Oh my! Any time ... ANY time."

Getting up from the bed, she tried desperately to relax but was feeling a whole other world of uncomfortable as her cervix responded to the invasion. Two days earlier a check had revealed she was 1 centimeter dilated, stretchy to 2 or 3, and 80% effaced. At the time this meant little to her. She knew she would need to dilate to "something the size of a bagel," but there was no tangible context, past or present, to understand the true process that was taking place in her body. This was her first child. The midwife understood but was reluctant to make any promises, so she only smiled and assured her that it would be "any time," as they said goodbye with a hug.

She was feeling terribly crampy and uncomfortable as she walked out the door and assumed it would settle on the way home, where she and her mother would continue making the chicken and salsa they'd started to prepare before the impromptu appointment with the midwife. Standing at the car, feeling too woozy and crampy too drive, she handed the keys to her mother and tried to get comfortable in the passenger seat, waiting for it all to pass. Back at home she gradually climbed the steep stairs up to her apartment and paused half way to breathe out the desperate cramping that was not subsiding. Once inside it began to dawn on her that there was a regularity to what was happening, an undeniable rhythm. She called her husband at work across the street asking him to come home. Hours earlier he had been so disappointed to wake to yet another day without the baby he was so anxious to meet. "Are you in labor?!" he asked when he heard her voice on the other end of the phone, she let go of her emotion and cried that she wasn't sure, but she was certain she needed him with her. Her mother stood in the kitchen looking excited and terrified all at once.

She had never imagined herself giving birth. Period. It was never on the radar. She and her partner of some 12 years had consciously decided to be "selfish" with their lives and that they would share their time together travelling, drinking wine, and seeking adventure, without the demands of infants that indefinitely grew into exacting toddlers and teenagers. She had gone so far as to dash her mother's only hope of becoming a grandmother when she told her, 7 months earlier, that they had decided to forgo children. Little did she know that within her body cell division was already performing its magic. When her breasts had hurt so much that she winced at the gentlest of hugs, and her regular period had been present but spotty, she bought a pregnancy test just to rule that unlikely possibility out before pursuing a visit to the doctor.

When her husband wandered into the washroom looked at the pee stick and called out, confused, "Is the blue line supposed to be there?" She was dumbfounded. Gobsmacked. Pregnant. They stood in separate rooms, shell-shocked for a moment before they found themselves together on the deck where he held her as she cried. They talked, though neither of them remembers what was said. They took the next few days to independently contemplate the information they'd just received. Termination was not out of the picture as they both worried they were not meant to be parents, and neither knew what the other truly wanted. It was he who suggested, two quiet days later, they not be afraid to embrace this new possibility, they were grownups after all, and she breathed a sigh of relief that he was brave enough to say it first. In an instant, they both grabbed on to the life growing inside of her and an invisible weight lifted from them as they raced for new information.

Now she found herself, 8 days past her estimated due date, likely in labor, pacing the hallway, anxious to see her husband walk through the door.

The contractions were more steady and insistent now, and when he arrived she reached out for his arms, held on to him tightly and connected with his eyes. Relief. Looking directly at him, taking deep breaths, she said "I can do this. I'm okay. I can do this," working more to convince herself it became her mantra and he became her talisman. When she was willing to admit that this was actually labor, she gave permission to call the midwife, and his mother who would travel in from an hour away. They would stay in their tiny one bedroom apartment above the bike shop, having made the decision to birth at home only days before – certainly not a consideration early in her pregnancy though her midwife had suggested how lovely it could be innocuously mentioning it at each of her appointments. Her husband would confess later that he had always hoped she would choose to have their baby at home but had never wanted her to feel pressured.

For her, giving birth at home was too unknown and frightening, she didn't know anyone who had done it, and her mother, who was normally quite silent on personal choices, would have none of it. But in the days before, as her due date came and went, the city hospitals had been in a state of SARS induced chaos and nothing was as it should be. During a late pregnancy visit to their home, the midwife had shown them what she would be wearing at the hospital so they wouldn't be alarmed when they saw her: safety glasses, surgical cap and gown, and a mask. She looked like she was entering a HazMat site, far from the colorful, confidence inspiring woman they had grown so accustomed to seeing. In hospital, women in labor were only permitted to have one support person present along with their midwife. Her husband would be the clear choice if that were the case, but she had planned to have the support of her mother and his mother, both women so vital in their lives, at the birth of their grandchild. Her mother had traveled from across the country to be there. When she called the hospital and had been told, in no uncertain terms, that there would be no exceptions to these new rules, she had cried fiercely as she felt her plans free fall from her grasp. He sat down beside her on the bed with his arm around her shoulder allowing her a moment to grieve before asking her "what do you want to do?"

That simple question stopped time and cleared any fear or doubt from her mind. She surprised herself when she answered that she wanted to have their baby at home, that she wanted to be surrounded by her family. He was happy to support her in this choice, and when she was grounded in her new certainty, they called the midwife to let her know. The midwife advised them to go and pick up the items that were listed in their prenatal kit for a homebirth. She arranged a shopping trip with her mother, returning home soon after with plastic sheets and extra towels.

The next night she began to feel what she was certain was the beginning of labor. The timing of the contractions were erratic, but they were stronger than the practice ones she had been feeling for the couple of weeks before. It was early evening and she suggested a walk to her husband, some final moments alone, hand in hand. She felt the strength of the surges increase as they walked, though they came sporadically and never lasted long. She was certain that this was the moment they had all so impatiently waited for. They headed back home to get some sleep; she knew that if labor was going to continue through the night she would need to get as much rest as possible while she could. She worried she would not be able to fall asleep and was surprised when she woke up briefly a few hours later still feeling her body working, but not distracting enough to prevent her from drifting off again.

When she awoke at 7:00 the next morning, she felt nothing. She waited. Nothing. When her husband opened his eyes and looked at her with frightened anticipation, she confessed to him that it had all stopped and that he should get ready for work. When she broke the news to her mother, it was hard to tell who was more disappointed. While he headed the few steps to work, she and her mother set off to run some errands and pass the dreary day. Throughout the day she felt nothing and began to entertain the idea that she may actually be the first woman to remain pregnant forever. Then the midwife called to say she had opening in her schedule, and with her mother they headed to the clinic.

It had only been two hours since she had stood in the midwives' office where the words "anytime now" had been spoken. Now, at home, and most certainly in labor, her midwife had arrived and was standing in her kitchen smiling. The midwife stood quietly and listened to her sounds and watched her move through the small apartment with the long hallway. She had found her rhythm and, eventually, with gentle assistance, a position that she would maintain for the remainder of her labor, standing and leaning back into her husband's arms as he supported her through each powerful surge and then falling slowly forward onto a stack of pillows that had been piled on the bed for her to rest on, her mantra of "I can do this" never leaving her head. Her mother in law arrived and shortly after came the student midwife. The three cats that resided in the apartment scooted to safer grounds – one cowering in the bedroom closet that would eventually emerge, looking petrified as the baby was about to be born and they would all freeze to allow him safe passage out.

She does not recall how she felt when the midwife quietly announced after her first vaginal exam that she was dilated 9 centimeters. She heard the muted voices of encouragement surrounding her, but she was in another place, following the definitive instruction she was receiving from her body. She knew she was being very vocal, but it felt good to "howl as the freight train was passing through" her body. She sent word to her mother, who was cutting rags and boiling water in the kitchen, that she was okay and not to worry. "Tell her I'm okay, please tell her I'm okay," she repeated to make sure the message was delivered. She intuitively understood how difficult it would be for her mother to hear the roaring sounds she was emitting with each contraction. The urge within her was unreal, like nothing she had ever imagined or felt before, it was all consuming but not painful. She likened it more to having an extreme bout of the flu and needing to urgently expel the contents of her body. She announced that she could feel the baby moving down, and 25 minutes later the midwife let her know that she was fully dilated and could begin to push when she felt like it. She shuffled to a more open area of the bedroom, still standing and leaning back into her husband's arms and chest, her legs wide, knees bent, lending her body to the increasing demand to expel, resting fully and completely in his arms in between the urges, eyes closed.

The midwives called for the two mothers in the kitchen to come for the birth, and the women eagerly and respectfully move into the room, choosing to sit at the head of the bed to witness the arrival of their grandchild. She is aware, somewhat, that they have come in, but she is getting tired from standing, and her quivering legs feel as though they are made of rubber. She does not know how far she has come or how far she has to go, only that it is happening and she has surrendered to it as completely as she can. She is not afraid but she wishes for it to be over, unsure of how much longer she can go on.

Her baby is crowning, and she can feel herself stretching an unfathomable and alarming amount. She has the clarity to remind the midwives that her husband would like to receive the baby, and he is directed out from behind to kneel at her feet, while the student steps into his place. Soon the midwife is asking her to slow down and not to push, an impossible directive to follow as her body is unstoppable, and she feels immense relief from the pressure as the baby's head is born. She hears her mother gasp in pure awe. The midwife reaches to remove a loop of cord from around the baby's neck and explains the normalcy of the procedure as she does, and then gently guides the father's hands to support his baby's head and waits. With the next contraction a chubby arm comes tumbling out followed by another, a torso, two legs and ten toes. The relief is instant but she still feels out of body. With the midwife's support, her husband lifts the baby up into her arms and resumes his position behind her encircling them both with his arms and whispers into her ear, "it's a girl." Again, his words have a clarifying effect and she takes in the babe she is holding, who has not yet cried. She remembers a woman from a birth video she watched talking to her baby as she waited for his first breath to come, and she does the same, greeting her daughter with a soft voice, "hi baby," letting her know she is home. The sound of her voice appears to bring a sporty cry from the new being, and the baby girl's skin grows pink. A breath of relief can be heard from the worried grandmothers who are hunkered on the bed. She is no small thing, this baby, and has a head chock full of dark hair. Later, after she has nursed and they've all had some time together, she will weigh in at a whopping 9 lbs 12 ozs!

For now, with this foreign yet familiar little creature in her arms, the newest mother in the room is helped over and onto the bed. Slowly she begins to notice her surroundings again, and the surrealness begins to abate. She has given birth. She's not sure what she expected, but it wasn't this. This is entirely other worldly. She feels like she has been conveyed through it all completely mystified. Now here she lay feeling a profound sense of gratitude with a near ten pound babe on her belly inching her way toward her breast. Her husband's eyes are damp, and she swears she can feel his heart swelling. Her mother cuts the cord with excitement as the student commits the memories to photographs. The midwife inspects and repairs her perineum, the swiftness of baby's arrival has caused a second degree tear but her euphoric exhaustion keeps her from caring or noticing much.

When it is done, she feels the power of her daughter's appetite as she latches for the first time. She is guided to the shower while he holds his daughter and the immediate flurry of birth settles while a new normalcy drifts into the little apartment. As the new family nestles in bed, staring at their combined creation, dear friends, who had waited faithfully nearby for the news, appear in the doorway with smiles and tears to congratulate them.

The midwives make their exit. The grandmothers take their turns holding their as yet nameless grandchild before leaving the new family for their first night together. They nestle her safely between the two of them and fall asleep staring at the incredible blessing that will change their lives forever for the better.

She doesn't believe she has ever felt anything akin to what she felt that night, the immense power of her body, the unconditional support and love of her family, the intuitive and ever trusting faith of her midwives. She knows she would never have imagined birth like this before, but now, she cannot imagine it any other way.

Perfection is Possible: Rising to the Challenge

by Hilary Monk

WITH MY FOURTH PREGNANCY, I was so afraid of the pain that was coming I used to cry whenever I thought of it because for me pain would never be enough reason to unnecessarily endanger the well-being of my baby by resorting to any kind of anesthesia. It got so bad that I sought out a therapist to help me deal with it. During the course of therapy, it was revealed that during the last birth I had been almost completely unsupported. All the wrong people were there, including somebody else's kids – not my own two – because the woman there to help with my children sent them away so she wouldn't miss the birth experience. During transition, which lasted five hours or so, my midwife went downstairs with my husband – SHE had to cry at MY pain – leaving me helplessly alone in the tub. She did not attend, she did not give me anything to drink from two o'clock in the morning until noon the next day, she was unprepared for the baby when he did make an appearance, and then she allowed me to be up nursing, cooking and serving breakfast to "my" birth team the morning after this twenty-four hour marathon. It had been so bad for me that I felt, mistakenly, that somehow I mysteriously sabotaged my next pregnancy, which I miscarried.

Once all this was out in the open, forgiveness for me and mine produced a new way; new possibilities were made available. I could, indeed, let go of all this, move into a space where my body was a friend, healthy and wise, where a different midwife, willing to work alone, would not distract from the relationship between my partner and me, where the experience could be joyful and private, where I could let go of every negative thought regarding outcome and process. This baby was the first to be anterior and deeply engaged at the onset of labor.

With a sense of gratitude, I embarked upon this labor – after a month or so of false labor that drove everyone crazy! – eighteen days postdates with no fear. When I went so far overdue, there was a minimum of fussing on my midwife's part. She knew what I wanted. We did our 'oxytocin challenge test' – stimulating my uterus by jumping up and down in her living room, giggling conspiratorially until a contraction came and then listening throughout with a fetoscope. It was the most intervention I would tolerate, and she was fine with that.

In early labor I went swimming in the local pool with my "baby" and his dad for the last time, stopping every so often to have a contraction. If the young man lifeguarding had known what was up, I can just hear it: "When's the baby due? ... "Oh, about two and a half weeks ago." ... "WHAT?" ... "and I'm in early labor right now."... "Not in my pool, you're not! Get the hell out, right now lady, or I'll ..." Come evening, the kids were sent away – and the labor stopped. So, to get things started my husband and I engaged in the most energetic sex we'd had since first meeting in our post-teens.

We went to bed at midnight, and at 1:00 a.m. I was literally kicked out of bed by a strong, beautiful contraction, and a few minutes later another, then another. I called my midwife to let her know, telling her it had just begun and to take her time. I labored for a while alone, walking the halls and grabbing the doorjamb to rock back and forth, consciously feeling grateful, excited, letting go of every fear-thought as it arose by picturing Ina May Gaskin, the author of *Spiritual Midwifery*, the book of birth stories that had inspired me to aim for natural labor at home, the most efficient and safest way to give birth in most cases. I gave myself over to my Higher Power with calming statements and patient glances, secure in the knowledge that birth works and is joyful. My midwife arrived unasked; we labored serenely together downstairs, walking, rocking on the nursing rocker; I gently declined the help she was eager to offer but which I really didn't need. Around 4:00 a.m. or so we went upstairs, woke my husband and checked me. I was about six centimeters and moving pretty well. As long as I relaxed and stayed open, there was very little pain – especially when I danced with my husband and kissed him to get things moving even more. He was amazing, looking deep into my eyes with every contraction, not a word. I could just about bite into his love and his breath as if into a ripe peach.

I labored some on my back, completely relaxed and joyous, except for one contraction where I tightened up, noted it, noted the pain with it, and said to myself, "I'm not doing another one like that, no way." The midwife, at my request, kept her fingers inside for a while – it felt s-o-o-o good – and suggested breaking the water. I asked what would happen, and she said, very seriously tongue-in-cheek, "Oh, nothing much. The baby will just come out." We all threw our heads back and howled with laughter at this. Then she explained very carefully what she was feeling and her reasoning around this, and only after securing my full agreement, she went ahead. The fluid felt warm and wonderful, but suddenly I was afraid for my baby – and said so. When she checked that the baby was doing great, I calmed right down. We decided to call my mum to bring the kids over soon.

Earlier, the midwife and I had discussed getting into some labor tincture to avoid the long drawn-out pattern of the previous birth, and she suggested it at this point. Labor tincture under the tongue – two good droppersful – and then WHAM! a huge contraction that pretty well knocked me mindless. The next twenty minutes are fuzzy for me – I recall squatting between two bodies holding me, being cradled between them, looking up after one contraction and laughing as if at a wonderful joke, saying, "God, I hate this part!" knowing full well the baby was coming really soon.

Shortly, I vaguely heard the kids come in downstairs. Then, at about 7:30 a.m., the weird bit happened – all adrenaline, no mind, part of the mind watching, amused, part terrified, mostly confused. My supporters talked me into sitting on the toilet in our teeny-tiny bathroom. I refused at first but couldn't articulate that it was because I knew that once I sat down, that was going to be it! And sure enough, the first contraction I had there was so enormous, the surge was so POWERFUL, so IMMENSE, so DOWN that my body tried to escape the force. The room was too small for me to stand and for my midwife to catch in front, so part of my mind, laughing all the while at the absurdity of it, watched as I stood up with the baby's head starting to crown. I watched myself put one foot up on the edge of the tub, the other onto the toilet seat, and reach overhead for the shower curtain rod to steady myself. My poor midwife was beseeching me, "What do you think you're doing? Come down!" but until the contraction ended I simply could not do anything but rise up. "I'm coming," I sang out as I descended with their help, the midwife crouching down and shuffling backwards before me with her hand under the baby's crowning head, my husband supporting me from behind. I zipped rapidly down the hall, way up on my toes with parted thighs to allow for the head there, reassuring the midwife that she was not, in fact, going to fall backwards down the stairs, and yelling over the banister, "Come, come, Mummy, hurry! Come on kids, you'll miss it!"

As we collapsed onto the bed in my room the rest of the baby's head gushed out, my husband catching with the midwife's guidance, and my kids all tumbled in one after another to stop, speechless, at the sight of their baby sibling emerging into their father's hands. I was distracted for only a moment as my baby birthed, calling out, "Look! Look!" to the kids, and then my mother who came in all rosy-faced with wonder at seeing her first birth. The baby was tiny and perfect, wiggling and squeaking from the word go, and I had to see right away (the midwife literally clamped her mouth tight shut as she already knew the baby's gender and knew the joy it would cause us) – a girl! after three sons, and especially after firmly coming to grips with accepting that she might be another boy after having lost a baby girl – I think – in the miscarriage the year before. My dad was there too, despite blood, placenta, baby, wetness, and all, and when I exclaimed that I was amazed at this, he said, "But of course I'm here!" and ruffled my hair, tears of joy leaking from his smiling eyes.

This birth was perfect, practically painless (I swore I'd never again feel too much pity for women whose babies were anterior, it was so easy) – and such ecstasy, such gratitude. All from prayer, from learning from past mistakes, from courage in the face of fear, from love and ease and certainty in the face of doubt.

Originally published as "Ecstatic Birth: According to Design." *Birth Gazette* (Fall, 1998), 14/4: 30-31.

♀ Breathing Under Water

by Sofie Weber

I can feel it getting colder. I don't care.
Drip – Patter – Patter
Drip
Drip
Patter – Patter
Drip
Drip
Breathe – Moan – Breathe – Clench – Drip – Drip
Drip
Holding On
Breathing Under Water

Hands are coming through the curtain but I can not open my eyes.
The rhythm of the water keeps me inside with you.
Breathe
Open
Open
Open – 8 – 9 – 10
Calling Out – Needing You – Only You – Come

I can't get out from under the waves. I've been here before.
Groaning – Grasping – Bearing – Trusting
Spinning
Pushing
Breathing
Screaming
Crowning
Pushing

Pausing
Almost here. I'm Consumed, Exhausted. Tears flow.
Focus!!!! Move!!! Breathe!!!!! Push!!!
Hold
Hold
Hold
Breathe
Calm
Breathe
Breathe
Cry

Embrace
Love
Remember

The Perfect Birth of Akadius

by Christa Niravong

MOTHERHOOD IS FULL OF GUILT. Even more so when you have the perfect birth. I feel guilty telling other mothers about my perfect birth experience with Akadius. It didn't start out so perfect because it was the night before the biggest contract our company had ever landed. We are self-employed. My husband, Frederick, and I had been working like crazy that month. We decided to ship our daughter Atarah off to Grandma for several days so that we could get our work done. As I was driving Atarah over to Grandma's place, I had started to feel some ever so light contractions, but I was in denial – there was so much work to do – and thought maybe they were just mild cramping.

I didn't want to believe that the birth would be tonight. It would be so inconvenient. Atarah and I read books and played together with Grandma's toys. I decided to take her to the park nearby. The cramps started to feel like contractions. Still, I denied it. We played at the playground and I was savoring this time with her.

She was so adorable. In fact, at two and half, I felt she had reached her peak of 'adorableness'. Everything about her was so wonderful. Her eloquence at such an early age, her physical acrobatic abilities, her sweet laugh. My heart burst with love for her and at the same time, mourned that this would be the last day we had together when she didn't have to share her parents. I had to sit down because the contractions were getting stronger. I saw the full moon in the dusky sky.

I finally conceded and called my doula to alert her at about 7:00 p.m. that I was going to birth tonight. I wobbled us back to Grandma's and took a shower. I had to admit to my mother-in-law that I had mild contractions but they were getting stronger. I knew I was going to deliver tonight. At 9:00 p.m., I called my husband to finish up his work. At 10:00, I tried to drive home, but fiddling with car seats took a while and we got home around 10:30 I was able to spend some precious moments with Atarah. She wanted to stay up a bit later, as if she could sense something was up. I nursed her to sleep and she finally went down at 12:30.

The contractions were strong enough to be convincing. I came downstairs and called my doula. Fifteen minutes later, I called the midwives. My doula arrived at 1:00 a.m. Nicole is a friend I had met through La Leche League and I had hired her as my doula because I really wanted someone there in case my husband was working. I had anticipated a precipitous birth and I didn't want just my two-year-old there to catch the baby. Nicole chatted with me. I got in our wooden bathtub. We chatted some more. She read my mind and gave me water to drink before I asked. The midwives arrived while I was soaking in my wooden tub. "Hey, welcome to the party."

A student midwife looked like she was not convinced I was in labor. I told them I ate beets for dinner so not to worry if I pooed red. They set up, I chatted more with my doula. She was a friend at my side. Then all four of us sat in my tiny bathroom and told stories and laughed between contractions.

Then, at one point, I had to focus. I chanted, "Welcome baby," while swaying my hips in the warm water and deep breathing. Even in transition, I felt I had breaks unlike in my first birth. I was calm and no one would have guessed that the baby was coming soon. I asked everyone to leave so I could defecate. I went back on the bed. I groaned a bit. Then I jumped up out of bed again because I had to urinate. Upon my return, I had an urge to push. I pushed. To everyone's surprise, my bag of waters shot across the room and hit the bookshelf, the wall, and the midwives. "That was satisfying," I said.

My doula ran up to get my resting husband (I wanted him to sleep so he would be prepared for the event that morning and so my daughter would have him by her side if she were to wake up in the middle of the night). My eyes were closed, I raised my right arm when I heard him enter the room, I interlaced my fingers with his strong ones. I pushed once, the head came out; I pushed the second time and felt the shoulders come out. It was 2:52 a.m. I was able to really feel the shape of the baby exit my body as it was a very satisfying and wonderful feeling.

Out came little baby X, who was nameless for two weeks or so. He wiggled his way up and breastfed. Lots of hair, cute little bum. The midwife asked if she could cut the cord since the blood had pulsed through ... so respectful of her to ask me. They never checked me or did anything that violated me in any way. My doula had really helped me understand and see the choices that I had. Midwives didn't need to examine me and check how dilated I was. They didn't weigh the baby right away or swing him around. I had quiet time with him and was able to savor these moments with him.

Six pounds, two ounces. My son. I don't remember him even crying when he came out. You would have to ask my doula if he did. She took some lovely non-invasive photographs. Calm little guy. I fell in love instantly. We slept skin on skin together. Daddy left for work on the biggest contract of our lives. I kept reminding myself that the money he made that one day would pay for the next year's expenses as well as post-partum care. I kept my post-partum doula for eight months. I learned that day that our baby was making a statement and reminding us that he didn't care about money. Also, he taught me to remember that people are important, and not things. What a lesson.

♀ Feeling All The Women

by Barbara Pal

Swirly fuzzy labor land
Intense, takes my breath away
Keep breathing through it

Pain and fear, intense sensations
Associated with trauma
Feels like I'm dying

The wave begins and
I get into rhythm
Be quiet and save your energy
Grrrr
Breathe breathe

Suddenly connection
Feeling other women
Time and space are fluid
We are all one

Ancient sisters birthing
On sand on rock
Some exuberant with life
Some dying
I feel them
Some births easy, some difficult
The same rhythm beats through us

Feeling other women now
We are laboring together now
Some who have done this before
Millions of us born this way
So that must mean I can do it

Young sisters up ahead
Not their turn yet but it will be
I know their surprise
Wanting to escape

In common is a pulse
Heart beating
Blood pumping
Umbilical placenta
A new life

A baby is born
A mother is born
Growing pains
Spiritual food
I feel them all
I feel us all
Circle of mothers
Warriors

Giving birth at home in 1970 Ontario

by Cady Williams

*Authors Note: In the late 1960s, I was part of a community of peo-
ple drawn together by the politics of social change. Most of us were
working as community organizers in Toronto, opposed the Viet
Nam War and inspired by people's liberation movements all over the
world. Some of us lived co-operatively, others in individual homes
close by. We discussed, questioned, researched, and experimented.
Young and consciously rebellious, we were eager to find new ways
to live and to effect change in what we experienced as a cold, profit-
driven, unjust world.*

Barbara Seaman's book, *The Doctor's Case against the Pill*,
appeared in 1969 and sent shock waves throughout the continent.
This was the first populist critique of the oral contraceptive pill.
The book revealed that women died in the first experiments with
the 10 mg pill, and that even the lower dose pill was causing dangerous side effects, such as blood clots and strokes. In 1968, I had
gone to the doctor everyone recommended to get the pill. Not yet
legal, a supply of the 4 mg oral contraceptives was handed to me
over his desk without question or a physical examination. A year

later, another doctor put me on a 2 mg pill (the dosage was decreasing that rapidly). Even on that dosage, I suffered a blood clot in my arm. One friend had a full blown false pregnancy. All of us were bloated but our periods were all but disappearing. What we had thought would bring us freedom to enjoy the so-called "Sexual Revolution" was actually making women ill and Seaman's book explained why. We stopped taking the pill.

We experimented with other forms of birth control, although the condom was not considered an option. One by one we became happily pregnant.

At first, we didn't plan to deliver at home. We researched pregnancy and birth and discussed hospital birth with women who had gone through that experience. In the hospital, it seemed birth was treated as an illness rather than one of life's everyday wonders. Women's birthing needs were not paramount. Women were lying on our backs, shaved, in stirrups. Fathers were not allowed into the delivery room. The valuable moisturizing and anti-bacterial protective vernix was washed off the baby immediately after birth. Babies were put in nurseries rather than rooming-in. We were exposed to germs we were not immune to. We did not want the cold, sterile, clinical atmosphere for our babies to greet the world.

The restrictions and culture of the hospital setting of that time drove us to consider other options. Neighbors who were medical students heard of our plans and gave us obstetrics textbooks, attempting to dissuade us by showing every strange anomaly that could be happening in our uterus and in labor. We had to find another source of information on natural labor and delivery. One of us found the British Midwives textbook – it contained the practical guidance that we needed.

At that time and for many years, Britain's birthing policy was that first births would take place in maternity hospitals and subsequent births, if not high risk, could be at home with the local Health Authority supplying a nurse midwife. With such a long history of practice, the textbook was the guide we needed and could trust.

There were a few doctors in Toronto who delivered at home. One of our friends chose this route because she lived in central

Toronto. Living outside the city, this was not an option for three of us. Visiting her and her baby after the birth strengthened my resolve to deliver at home. It was the warmth and comfort that most impressed me. The mother was calm and relaxed speaking about the birth. I listened to a most ordinary yet extraordinary story. Among the many remarkable aspects of their birth experience was the blending of the placenta into a smoothie, which both mother and father drank. When my son was born several months later, my partner and I contemplated doing this, but by the time we were ready, the day after the birth, the placenta had disintegrated. We buried it in the vegetable garden.

We had doctors, who, while trying to dissuade us, agreed we were healthy, showed no discernible risk factors, were well versed on pregnancy, and knew when to head to a hospital if complications arose. They agreed to meet us at the local hospital if it became necessary.

We got this somewhat reluctant cooperation even though home birth was technically "allegal" – outside statutes and common law concerning birth. We knew officially we would have to say that it all happened so fast that we could not make it to a hospital. We were lucky that no one turned us in, or perhaps it was a sign of the times that people trying new approaches to life were becoming accepted.

Our families were not told of our decision. We needed to create the space to do what we planned without having to deal with questions or worry, to experience our journey without any doubt. They were told after the fact when the focus became our healthy babies.

Grantley Dick Read's *Childbirth Without Fear*, and Marjorie Karmel's, *Thank You Dr. Lamaze* were the only books we found on how to deal with labor. We picked the Lamaze method because we found the techniques helpful and focused on what was happening in our bodies. The method incorporated the father into the birthing experience. We practiced the breathing and relaxation techniques together following the instructions in the book, preparing to let our bodies do the work.

On my due date, my partner and I went to a friend's home to await the babe's arrival. We understood that the concept of a due date was far too mathematical to indicate what was happening in a pregnant woman's body, but still we started the vigil on that day and every morning she was greeted by expectant looks to which she would shake her head. Not surprisingly, this became an annoyance to her as the wait lasted two weeks.

When it did begin, the labor went through the night and the contractions followed no discernible pattern. Two minutes, break, then one, then five, then seconds. Short contractions, then very long ones. The big fireplace was burning bright and beautiful in the darkened room. It was a moving and primal scene with her breathing and she and the dad working together. We sat, my partner and I, witnessing and giving aid when needed, keeping the fire going. I shot photos and fed her. The sac appeared and the dad got excited that the baby would come out in it (we had read this was a good omen). "Break it!" she called out and a wonderful relieving groan came as the fluid flowed. Soon, she squatted, pushed and delivered a baby girl so thickly covered with the white creamy vernix that she looked like a living statue. It was absorbed within a half hour of her birth and we all got to soak in some ourselves as we held her.

At first, for a second, the baby was still. Then the pink and the cry and after the mother fell back in relief from the delivery, she leaned up and reached her arms for her daughter. The photo I took of that moment became a centrefold in a Toronto underground newspaper, *Harbinger*. Birth as centrefold. Real nudity in the real world. A touché to the Playboy centrefolds that objectified women so egregiously.

Four months later, my son was born. I ignored the due date, not wanting to have the pressure of a vigil. The day before labor began, I went for a walk down the country road lined with black-eyed susans and felt heavy for the first time. I had wanted to deliver under the willow tree in front of the house, but it was a dull and drizzly day, so I labored and gave birth in our bed of yoga mats on the floor, so most of the room was the birth bed.

As in the first birth, our medical student friends had given us a blood pressure monitor but also a sterile package we were to open when I went into labor. We all burst into laughter when we found draping for my body including one with a hole through which the baby would be born.

My brother-in-law, a photographer and artist, was behind the camera, and none of the photos turned out because he had been so mesmerized by what he was seeing through the lens that he forgot to take light meter readings.

It was a textbook first birth with gradual intensity and spacing of contractions. My partner massaged my back, I breathed, talking to my body throughout, urging on the contractions.

In transition I learned about the difference between real pain and labor "pain"; about the consequences of handing over direction to another; about leaving my body and having my logical mind take over and losing the rhythm of what had been a great labor up until then.

My partner checked me and (over) confidently declared I was 10 centimeters dilated. I heard instructions to push coming from outside of me. I obeyed rather than listening and staying with myself. With this artificial push, I screamed in excruciating pain, felt myself leap into the air. This was pain. Labor contractions were something else. I had pushed too soon and had to go back before I could go ahead to deliver. I still use this example when talking about labor and pain. I still think we haven't found the right descriptive word for what we experience. "Surge" doesn't do it for me. A client thinks "earthquake" fits.

My most wonderful memory was when my son was about to come out of me. We understood that one of the reasons a woman can tear in delivery is that the pressure around the vaginal opening is uneven if she is not in a good position. In squatting, the pressure was uneven and the position uncomfortable. Then I knelt, leaning forward with my arms around the necks of my partner and another dad. The wonderful part was that I could look down, see my son's head come out and watch him, knowing exactly what to do, turning his head. My son slid out of me, fully pink and giving out loud yells rather than baby cries. I later thought perhaps he was angry that his progress and work had been interrupted by that earlier disruptive push.

Born in the bed and we stayed in that bed. I lay awake all night looking at this new and glorious human.

When we decided to register our son's birth, we had two people arrive from the registry office to help us – and them – fill out the forms. They had not had a birth in the township since the 1930s.

The third birth was unexpectedly different. After several days of the birthing mother walking outside in the summer sun and occasionally stopping to rub her belly with a big smile on her face as she had a contraction, she went into a short, intense labour and within a few hours, was pushing. No overnight or all day experience for her and us all. We quickly adjusted and gathered closer to help.

When I came into the birth room, my body was enveloped with the smell, sounds, the air of birthing. I could feel exactly what she was going through. I sat with her, holding my 5-week-old son who lay so calmly, with a look of awe on his face, his eyes wide open and his mouth quietly opening and closing. He looked like he knew where we were as well as what was happening.

This baby girl came fast, with the cord wrapped around her neck and the dad deftly slipping it off but lost some control of the speed of her delivery. The mother had a small perineal tear, which she only noticed the next day. There had been no massive bleeding as we had been warned would happen if any of us tore. We took her to the hospital to be stitched up and received surprised and cool reception from the nurses.

We weren't the only ones who had chosen to deliver at home without a medical professional. CBC Radio recognized this and did a program with my partner and I and several other couples who had chosen this path.

We helped each other through the first months of parenting but then gradually as our partnerships and marriages disintegrated, we lost track of each other. We moved on in our lives, taking new directions after we had taken leave of these relationships.

My path followed that of my son's as a single parent. I chose cooperative living situations so he could grow up with other children, was involved in developing day care and later an alternative school. At the same time, I maintained my involvement in women's health issues: witnessing births and helping postpartum; learning more about the long-term effects of the birth control pill especially as it relates to cancer; and working on other reproductive issues such as healthy forms of birth control and abortion rights.

After years of non-partisan and partisan political organizing work and a variety of jobs to fund my activism, I am now studying and practicing to be a doula, I am both heartened and shocked the more I learn. Heartened by pregnant women and their partners determined to have the births they want, by those who have developed the midwife and doula movements, by the advancement in natural laboring and delivery techniques, and by the research done by doctors, midwives and doulas that reveals the problems and offer solutions. Shocked by the impatient attitude toward the onset of labor, with due dates having an unsubstantiated and illogical strength and induction of labor being the norm rather than the exception; by the stunningly high cesarean rate; by, in general, the lack of progress toward women-centred birth in hospitals.

I have stopped at the farmhouse where my son was born. I have also gone with my son on his birthday. The house is barely standing and with the road expanded, there are no longer ditches with black-eyed susans. It will always be a sacred place for me and yet perhaps many more were born there when home births were the norm. I want to put up a memorial plaque but then that would commemorate the birth as unique and historic rather than another one of life's everyday wonders.

Being in the Birthing Field

by Crescence Krueger in Conversation with Elena Tonetti-Vladimirova

"WE ARE WHAT WE BELIEVE WE ARE." Elena Tonetti is a master of the imagination. You may know of her through her documentary film, *Birth As We Know It*, released in 2006. It is a testament to the clear, calm power a woman is able to access when she gives birth free of fear. The film includes footage of women giving birth in the Black Sea in the 1980s and more recent footage of an orgasmic birth shot in Hawaii. Elena played a key role in these events. She has been a revolutionary force in changing what we imagine is possible for ourselves and our children.

Born in Russia, Elena initially trained as an actor and worked in the theatre. An actor's instrument is her own body and mind; her skill lies in her ability to transform them. Since giving birth is the ultimate act of transformation, Elena had a good foundation for the groundbreaking birth work she would later become a part of. First, though, she was involved in social and political transformation. Through "Citizen Diplomacy" she took part in an underground movement to end the Cold War, and with her late husband she facilitated large events called 'Games'– they reworked the power structures of civic and business institutions and were a catalyst to significant economic change in the USSR. In 1982, Elena was introduced to Igor Charkovsky. A pioneer in water birth, Igor had a vision of changing society at its source through peaceful, conscious birth. Elena offered to use the skills and human infrastructure she had developed in the 'Games' to promote his vision. Within a year, it had manifested as a real social movement and a camp was set up at the Black Sea where selected women gave birth in the warm, shallow waters.

In her film Elena says, "When love, not fear, is an integral part of the birthing field, a woman has access to the power of creation that is working through her. The more power is in her field, the less force she will need to use because Life is ... highly coherent." Life is intelligent. It is also mysterious. I found Elena to be the same! After taking part in one of her workshops here in Toronto, I met with her at the home of a mutual friend. Elena and I ended up talking in the room that Natalia had given birth in a year or so earlier. I had been a part of the birth and my return to the room with Elena seemed to set the tone for our conversation, taking us into a timeless place. As Elena told me about her life, I felt like she was weaving a fairy tale. She spoke of a grandmother who sent her out into the woods alone, marriages, a shaman, a tight rope walker, the fall of the iron curtain, a lagoon, Mecca, swimming babies, and wild dolphins. In the end, it was a tale of a woman coming to terms with her own life, her own power, a tale of a woman giving birth to herself. Here's some of the telling of it!

Crescence Krueger One of the things I got out of your workshop was that we define ourselves by our stories. Traumatic birth stories limit our idea of what is possible. With you, we re-imagined the story of our own birth. We liberated our imagination. And this is the first step to freedom, isn't it? Birth starts in the imagination and the arc of a birth story is the journey, for many people, from a state of fear to a state of love. When you were with women giving birth in the Black Sea, hours away from medical support, that trajectory had to be there for them. How did you work with women so that they were in love when they gave birth?

Elena Tonetti-Vladimirova How much time do we have for this? [laughter]

CK Natalia invited me for dinner ... so it's up to you!

ETV Uh huh. [laughter] All right. Yeah, it's a very big subject because it's true that we are what we believe we are. We are what we remember about ourselves, what we allow ourselves to be. We are the product of our own ideas about ourselves. And when society doesn't have positive role models of good birth, then bad births are all we have, basically. So ... to overcome this inertia ... it's nothing other than inertia because really, any cat knows how to give birth. There's nothing extraordinary about giving birth, just like there's nothing extraordinary about any process of elimination. All of our functions of eliminating stuff that is ready to be eliminated are built into the perfect design of our bodies. It's our belief that we need intervention to give birth that causes most of the complications. It's important to understand first that the birthing field is the field of pure potentiality. That is how not only every living form is created but how universes are created, stars and ah ... everything that we see. You know it is first an idea, some kind of notion, some kind of, some kind of speck of consciousness, and then everything else starts building up around that speck. Same with a human baby. So if we allow ourselves to understand the experience of people making, if we open our psyche and our nervous system to viewing making a baby as something more than a mechanical, physiological process, this is where we start, in a place of potential.

CK What gets in the way of a woman realizing her potential?

ETV Well, a woman needs to neutralize her own birth trauma. That's number one requirement in overcoming the limitations of inertia. Number two, if her husband is present, he needs to neutralize his birth trauma. Then number three, we need to do this with every single person who will be present, including the parents, siblings, medical delivery team, if they are present, midwives and doulas and friends. If anybody is present who has not dealt with their own birth trauma, their anxiety will inevitably affect the field, the presence. Their anxiety affects it just the way radiation affects the environment. It's not seen; it cannot even be tasted or smelled; it's just this omnipresent…

CK But it's so tangible…

ETV Yeah. It's that omnipresent feeling. It's the energy of the counter intention to being alive, to being in the body, and the counter intention to being alive is very powerful. I think it's the most common cause of death. [laughter] It's that death urge that we acquire from the first breath or even from inside the mother's womb. When the environment doesn't feel safe and friendly and we start doubting the original intention of our spirit to be in a body, we say, "Yikes! Maybe I'm not meant to be here. Maybe I should go back!" But the Life force is very powerful so it keeps building itself, building the body and the breath, and we come into the world. But it doesn't mean that there's a sense of safety, and that indecisiveness about whether we want to be alive or not is a very powerful counter-intention to getting anything done, never mind giving birth to a baby. So if we are in the position of making a new person, we better get on board with the situation and just [sigh] … be present for it and agree to be in our body. This is the thing: the mother first of all has to come to terms with her own life, with her own ownership of the body.

CK And how did you help women do that?

ETV It changed over the years. When I started in Russia, we used a lot of ice swimming. The effect is very powerful when you go for a few seconds in ice cold water, not just the cold shower, but the kind where you have to break the ice with an axe first and then you jump in. It's so cold it feels hot! It just burns your skin, it's so cold. In winter, that's what Russian people used to do traditionally. We used that extreme sensation to really learn to be present in the body instead of freaking out, instead of screaming and trying to get out of it. We used that intensity in order to find a way to completely relax into it. There is something very magical about it. You feel like a newborn. You really feel something's shifted. It's a very powerful experience. And it was never done for any length of time. You know, you don't get in that ice cold water and just sit there. You jump in and out. It's very short. Unless you're pregnant. Pregnant women used to [laughter] ... they used to just swim and swim and swim [laughter].

CK Because they had a warm little life inside!

ETV Yeah! Everybody else did all sorts of warm-up exercises and then they jumped in and jumped out, bright red, and got dressed really quickly! But the pregnant women, they strolled in, undressed, got in the water ... [laughter] You know, it's like they were on a completely different planet.

CK And was that a traditional Russian thing for pregnant women to do?

ETV No. That started only with our conscious procreation movement in the 1980s. It was never advised for pregnant women to do that traditionally. You know, the people didn't have a very good survival track record. If a woman had 20 children, she might keep five or six of them. Children died at a very high rate, so people were trained to eliminate anything that might trigger illness. But we found the ice swimming to be a very helpful mechanism. And then our way for years in Russia was also the psychic healing because the person who discovered water birthing, Igor Charkovsky, he was ... well still is ... a very powerful seer and ... he is a shaman. There is no way not to say this. [laughter] That's what he is. That's how he came up with this concept of water birth in the first place, seeing it in his visions and understanding that that's what would be good for people, to incorporate water into the birth process. In his healing sessions with pregnant women he would see how a woman's mother could be the cause of her complications during her pregnancy, or a woman's grandmother. Or even her grandmother's grandmother. He went into generations and generations of very complex interplay within the family lineage. When he would clear the energy connections – he used to call them cords – when he would disconnect those cords and free a woman from all the baggage that was handed to her by her mother and all the older women in her family, all of a sudden, the symptoms that she was having during pregnancy would disappear. Instantly. That was quite a powerful experience because at that time there was absolutely no concept of prenatal psychology in the mass mentality. It was early 1980s. We heard nothing from the West, and even the American Association of Prenatal Psychology was just barely forming and the research had not yet been published, never mind translated into Russian, so we had no way of reading all that stuff that is available now on the Internet. Now you can find a huge body of research in this field. But at that time, it was just Igor who was telling us. So what we had for a long time was just winter swimming and Igor doing his sessions. Then from the West came the notion of re-birthing and the notion that the woman's own birth trauma played into the symptoms that she was having. So we started doing lots of re-birthing.

CK And what did that involve?

ETV Re-birthing was a very specific, intense breathing technique with a specific intention to allow people to experience their own original birth. And because there had usually been a lot of trauma involved in their birth, the re-birthing would be very cathartic, lots of screaming and yelling and people would remember exactly how they had gotten hurt and how much they had gotten hurt and how scared and terrified they had been. It was always extremely dramatic and that was not really very effective. Years after trying to incorporate re-birthing, I noticed that people remained symptomatic no matter how many sessions they did. It didn't seem like it was going anywhere, so I looked for a way to replace that technique.

Instead of reinforcing the trauma and feeding the original birth trauma even more ... when we think about something and give it our attention and our undivided energy, it just feeds it and it becomes even stronger and has a more powerful hold on our system ... I came up with the process that I call 'Limbic Imprint Recoding'. I hold the space for a group of people to go through steps that involve specific breathing and movement that allows them to go into a slightly altered state of being. In this state they create their own new experience of being conceived and gestated and born. I noticed how much healing happened when people acquired a new reference point instead of reinforcing what had originally happened. And I noticed that for people who were fighting infertility, they were able to conceive right after going through this process because the inability to conceive has something to do with that counter intention to being alive.

CK Well, to be able to conceive a thought...

ETV Right. Right.

CK Conceive of something...

ETV Right.

CK Yeah, so it's that limit of imagination.

ETV Right. See that's the thing, a woman might think that she wants a baby but her body is not on the same page. Her body is freaking out at the thought of the invasion by some other being. Her thought and her body's feeling are in completely different areas of the brain.

CK Do you want to talk more about that because for me it was a new understanding about the limbic brain and how when we're babies and small children, our cortex hasn't developed enough to be able to link to it?

ETV Yeah. So for example, if a woman who can't conceive thinks that she wants to have a baby, her thinking is happening in the cortex. But inability to conceive is happening in her reptilian brain, which is the part of the brain on top of the spinal cord that is responsible for our pure physiology, the physiological processes of being alive. That's the part of the brain that is responsible for a person being considered alive when they are in a coma, for example. There is no thinking. There are no feelings. But the physiology is still pulsating and functioning; it's governed by our reptilian brain. This part of the brain is also the catalyst to the physiological process of conceiving a baby. So we need to get to that part of our being where we can allow ourselves to create that original cosmic, ecstatic explosion that divides the egg in the first place to start forming the baby's body. For that to happen, the woman needs to recognize him and open herself to him, fall in love with him, so to speak, her knight in shiny sperm armor. There is nothing short of a miracle in that event. The membrane of the cell we call 'the egg' is the most impenetrable wall in this three-dimensional world. It's the largest cell in the body and is most protected from anything that might disturb it. The sperm is the smallest, very disposable and vulnerable cell. How is he supposed to get in?! His tail is only strong enough to keep him going the full length of his Odyssean journey to find her, and usually by the time he gets there, his resources are quite spent. He is not equipped with anything to conquer the bastion! With all the immense knowledge that modern science has acquired about this moment, there is no scientific explanation of it, only observations about what it looks like at every stage. *Nothing* about how it actually works and why it doesn't work when it doesn't. I believe that for answers we need to look at a bigger picture than what the three-dimensional vision offers. And the pathway to that magic is through the self organizing, creative vortex of the Birthing Field. It is like a shamanic portal that allows something that did not exist to come into being. The key to that portal lies within the realm of our limbic system of the brain, not through the cortex. The limbic brain is where our feelings, senses, emotions, ability to love, or inability to love are governed from. It is the home of our ability to remember our spirit's intention for being in the body. The limbic brain is the common ground where our cortex (mind, the thinking organ) can connect with our physiology (the reptilian brain). So the limbic imprinting that happens at birth (from the moment of conception through gestation, birth and the first few years of life) is the same mechanism that programs the 'basic settings' in our nervous system in matters regarding our emotional life ... Have you seen *The March of the Penguins?*

CK I haven't.

ETV No? It shows this amazing drive the species has. They march for months through snow, through storm, through dreadful conditions. They march and march and march to a specific place to lay an egg. And then they march for months, the females, they march to another place, miles and miles away, to eat. And it doesn't occur to them that they could just go and have babies where they can eat.

CK Because it's their imprint to march?

ETV Yeah, they go through unbelievable drama and some of them die. Their life is spent covering an enormous amount of territory. Because they don't have a developed cortex, they can't ask, "Why can't we just live where we can both eat and have our babies? The drive to march is happening in their limbic brain and they don't have the capacity to question it.

CK So we're like penguins.

ETV When we live according to the narrow corridor of our comfort zone, we are. We have a very narrow range of experience that our nervous system translates as what's comfortable, what's good. If a baby is born into suffering, suffering becomes its comfort zone. If the baby experienced aggression, abandonment, loneliness, then that's what she will experience as her comfort zone throughout her life, unless she decides to break that habit and acquire a new good habit in which something other than suffering is interpreted by the nervous system as comforting. So it's a very tricky thing. People have deliberately used this mechanism on animals for thousands of years. If you tie a baby elephant to a stick in the yard, that baby will rage for about a week and then it will give up and live being tied to a stick on a chain. A year later, you can pull that stick up and the elephant just stays put. No thought comes through about being able to leave. The possibility of going back to jungle doesn't cross its mind. That is the way that people have trained camels and horses and bears in the circus and lots of other mammals, including humans. That is how for thousands of years, thousands, people have created slaves and soldiers.

CK Michel Odent speaks about that. He says not giving the baby colostrum and not giving the baby the breast creates an absence of love.

ETV And then in the absence of love, it's very easy to manipulate a person and make them kill people, or serve, or be a robot basically.

CK Which is why this work is revolutionary. You said that you came to realize that political transformation wasn't getting to the root of what our societies really need, that the root is in birth and childhood. Was that a conscious transition for you from politics to birth?

ETV Oh yeah! When I started working with Igor Charkovsky, I was the last person to get involved in birthing because I wasn't going to have any babies! My own birth trauma was so tremendous and traumatic that I made a decision very early in life not to have my own babies and to do everything I could to prevent my friends from having babies. I was very clear that multiplying misery was not a virtue and that we just needed to cut the crap, so to speak. "Stop creating more people!" That was my idea of reducing the amount of suffering on this planet.

CK So how did the transition into birth work come about for you?

ETV I was involved with my late husband in something called 'Games'. We were creating oases of common sense in the way our society was functioning, finding solutions to seemingly unsolvable problems. We played 'Games' with the City Council of Moscow, with nuclear stations, with the Ministry of Transportation ... At the end of each 'Games' session, the organization would develop a very clear, step by step, plan of action about how to get out of the deep doo they were in! At that time in Russia, every level of the economy was falling apart and everything was in such bad shape that every organization needed something like that. By the time my husband stopped ... he got very ill because it was just inhumane to process that much energy ... we had a waiting list for the 'Games' of six years ahead. My introduction to Igor Charkovsky was to see if I could get our 'Games' team involved with his project. He had been working for 20 years and was not getting anywhere. He had only done something like six births by the time I got involved in 1982. Igor explained the whole concept of prenatal psychology, how the way we are born affects the quality of our life and how all the mess in Russia was the result of our inability to thrive as a society and as individuals. He said the concept of thriving was removed from each person at birth. He said the expectation of our needs not being met was tied into the practice of babies being taken away from their mothers for five days after they were born and that the inability of Russian people to come together and work together to solve their problems was rooted in their early experiences of life. He was able to convince us to drop everything and start working with him. And all of a sudden, it was very clear to me that unless we started making new people without them being harmed, we would be recreating in geometrical proportions the mess we were already in. Within the first year of our work, there were classes all over Moscow and it became a whole social movement. Thousands of people wanted to have an alternative to the conventional Soviet State Birth House. There, women were treated like criminals. They were abused, hit, and called names and treated like they'd done something bad by getting pregnant, you know. It was really not a nice place.

CK Was it the severity of the hospital environment that pushed people to move toward an alternative? Here in Canada there seems to be more inertia now, I think, than there was 20 or 30 years ago when feminism took birth on as an issue. Feminism doesn't seem to be a relevant concept for the younger generation now. And technological intervention has increased even more and so the caesarean rate is increasing ... we're now at 30% ... the thought of thousands of people taking courses in how to give birth naturally, I just don't see that happening here. Why did it happen in Russia?

ETV Well, the number one driving factor was the severity...

CK It was just so awful.

ETV Yeah, it was just so awful that it was a "no-brainer" to try something else. And it was a different atmosphere. The Cold War was melting and the shift was dramatic. Earth-bound spirituality was budding. Women were searching for ways to connect with the core of Life. So it was time for this idea. Nothing is more powerful than an idea whose time has come and I just happened to be in the right place at the right time and I surfed that wave. And had a blast surfing it too, you know? It was really, really awesome what was happening, really exciting and empowering and just an amazing experience. I also think that we were a generation of people who were not drugged. Drugs were available to only a very few members of a privileged layer of Russian society...

CK Drugs?

ETV Drugs in birth. So many of the mothers who are pregnant now were drugged at birth. So their understanding of birth is ... absent. They don't know anything about giving birth because they don't know anything about being born. That's another big piece: a woman knows about giving birth by being born. She receives every bit of information necessary by going through the birth canal. And if a drug is introduced, or any kind of extreme sensory overload, especially caesarean section, circumcision etc., that part of their nervous system is never activated; and their birthright, the full scope of their abilities might remain dormant. Lots of our capacities require specific activation. You know, we don't need to read books about how to poop, for example. But we need to have that experience in order to know how to poop. Or how to eat. Our ability to do something...

CK Neurologically, we need to go through the experience.

ETV Yeah. And the knowledge of how to give birth is one of those things that needs to be activated. The design is there. The anatomy and the neurobiological blueprint is there, but it needs to be activated. If a woman did not go through being born properly, that piece is not activated and so when she finds out that she is pregnant, she freaks out.

CK Her limbic imprint is either damaged, incomplete or it hasn't fully manifested.

ETV Right. It's not there. When I was little, my parents would send me to our dacha, our country house. Almost every Russian family had a house in a village somewhere in the country.

CK Like a cottage.

ETV Like a cottage, yeah, where kids were sent with grandmothers to spend all three months of summer vacation. And my grandmother would send me into the forest with a jar to pick berries. It was a big jar and I hated it. [laughter] Hated it! All day! It would take me all day to find enough berries and so I had a lot of adventures. Imagine a little girl with a big jar wandering in the forest all day! I ran into quite a lot of things that I experienced as activation of different abilities and capacities. For example, when she sent me in the beginning, I would say, "What if I get lost?" I whined and tried to get out of it and I remember … it's like 50 years later … I remember her saying, "What, are you stupid? Why would you get lost? You know how to find your way home!" And of course I wouldn't think, "Yeah I'm stupid." No! So my grandmother, just by this one sentence, she activated my sense of direction. I knew how to find home because my grandmother told me I would.

CK She expected you to come home.

ETV Yeah.

CK And so you did.

ETV Right. I didn't know that I had that knowledge in me. But she said I did. So I came home.

CK Whereas, if she had said, "Now, don't get lost Elena!"

ETV Right! Exactly. Getting lost was not an option. She was so matter of fact. There was no big deal about it. She activated a completely different level of responsibility in me. "I'm paying attention because I'm smart." My grandmother delivered that piece of information just like that! [snaps her fingers]

CK We expect to get lost in birth.

ETV In birth, we don't know that we're not stupid, that's the thing. [sigh]

CK Did you take that faith in our innate intelligence with you to the Black Sea? How did you all feel safe to have births there?

ETV Well, here is a story that describes our basic attitude. We had a woman who was a tight rope walker in the circus and I asked her, "How do you do it? What happens when there's no net?" And she said, "Oh, when there is no net, we don't fall." It's a powerful metaphor for birth. When a woman knows that it's up to her, it's a very different level of responsibility that she carries and a different level of concentration ... of digging deep. At the Black Sea, it was not a "come on everybody" situation. We hand picked the couples. It was our joke that this was the Russian Olympic Birthing Team. Doctors and midwives were not allowed. Anybody who went through medical school and was contaminated by pictures of pathology, there were no such people. None of us had any formal medical education and we had no complications.

CK You hadn't imagined them.

ETV No. They were not an option. There were some labors that went longer than the others, but that was it. Maybe a birth was longer, but then the baby came out and everybody was happy and we feasted on placenta fried with garlic and onion. And salt. That was the most delicious meal in the whole world because there were no refrigerators there. There was no electricity. We were just living on produce, you know ... [laughter] ... salads and fruits and vegetables because you couldn't have any dairy. The group of organizers camped there all summer. It was this shallow lagoon that was quite a bit of a hike to get to. It's hard to tell now how long it was because I was very young and it felt like nothing. It was just a beautiful walk along the trail. It wasn't on the beach; it was actually a goat trail on the cliff with a hike down on a very steep hillside, mountainside. When I look at pictures of the camp now, I think, "Oh my God!" We were so naïve! I have no idea what we were thinking. We were young, naïve, and idealistic. I don't know, I want to say stupid but ... I don't think we were stupid; we were just so completely in the bubble of ... it was on the verge of being stupid ... but see, we got away with it.

CK Stupidity with a higher purpose maybe?

ETV Yeah. It was not about risking our lives. It was about our spiritual practice. It was the equivalent of a monastery. That birthing lagoon was our Mecca. It was protected by the most incredible wings of ... I don't know, we were not ... raised in religion. We only vaguely knew who Jesus Christ or God was because there was no religious education. Communism was atheistic religion. So we did not pray to gods or angels or ... we did not have that sort of imposed religion, but we all were deeply spiritual people.

CK I'm guessing you tapped into your own organic...

ETV Into our own. We created our own gods and ideas of how to connect with the Source without being imposed upon...

CK So it was true. It was authentic.

ETV It was. Absolutely.

CK It wasn't dogma.

ETV Yeah!

CK Yeah.

ETV Everyone found their own specific flavor of how they were meditating, how they were praying. We used the words "meditation" and "prayer" that we knew from western religion and eastern religion but because nobody really knew what they were, everyone came up with what worked for them. And it was the most direct experience of connection with the Source that people can possibly have.

CK Yeah.

ETV You know, it was very beautiful. It was so pure and so innocent. Being in the field of that birthing lagoon, everyone felt completely safe. There were no accidents. I believe that we can create a happy humankind in the next 20 to 30 years, if we learn to respect the newborn's rights and welcome the new generation properly, without traumatizing them with unnecessary suffering due to our lack of knowledgeable role models. Babies are deeply feeling people and their experiences are recorded in their flesh and bones. It is up to us to set the stage right for them.

Elena's website is www.birthintobeing.com

Birth in 1983

by Deborah da Silva

AT 4:50 P.M. ON TUESDAY, NOVEMBER 22, 1983, I awoke suddenly from an afternoon nap with a feeling of wetness. I realized my water broke. After the initial shock of realizing that I was going into labor and would finally be having my first baby, I called my husband Al at 5:00 p.m. He left work immediately and came home. While I was waiting for him to come home, I washed my sweat pants and underwear, packed a few more things for my suitcase to go to the hospital. Ten minutes after my water broke, I began to have mild contractions. When Al came home he got ready, had a bite to eat, and made a sandwich for the hospital. Shortly afterwards, we left for the hospital.

I was admitted to the hospital at 7:00 p.m. After answering several dozen questions, I was taken to the labor room where I was given a shave and enema. (Remember, this is 1983.) The nurse checked to see how far my cervix was dilated, which was less than 1 centimetre. At 7:50 p.m. Al was allowed in the labor room. A nurse came in and gave me a square flat pill: "The doctor wants you to take this". Upon inquiring what this pill was, I was told it was to make my contractions come along faster. I took it but felt I should have been given a better explanation.

My contractions were approximately 1 minute long and about 8 minutes apart. I used the slow chest breathing I learned at Lamaze class and found it fairly easy to relax. I was able to read and crochet, but occasionally I would have the urge to go to the washroom to get rid of everything inside of my colon from the enema. This was a real nuisance because it seemed to me that every time I went to the washroom I would have one contraction after another and it was difficult to relax. I had nothing to focus on to help relax me.

At 10:30 p.m. my contractions were about 45 to 60 seconds long and 1 1/2 to 2 minutes apart. I could not read or crochet. I found the shallow breathing most useful at this point. The nursing staff would come in occasionally and check the baby's heartbeat, which meant I had to get into bed. After they finished, it was very painful to get out of bed, but I had to because my contractions seemed worse in bed. I spent most of my labor in a rocking chair.

At 11:30 p.m. the doctor came in to check how far I was dilated. He said to the nurse "she's three fingers" and then got up and left without saying a word to me. The nurse told me that I was half way to being fully dilated.

At 12:00 p.m., my contractions were 1 1/2 minutes long and 2 minutes apart, although the time between contractions varied. I was using the transition breathing at this point, although I didn't realize I was in transition. Al was very helpful because he helped me slow down my breathing, which helped me to relax. My contractions peaked very quickly and were very strong to unbearable. It was at this point I asked Al to get the nurse because I wanted something for the pain. He tried to convince me that I was being psyched out because I could hear women being rolled down the corridor to the delivery room that were moaning and groaning very loudly.

I was beginning to feel sick. Al finally got the nurse who was going to give me Demerol to relax me. At 12:20 a.m., I got into bed and vomited the Jell-O I ate before I came to the hospital. I felt much better. At 12:25 a.m. the nurse gave me the shot of Demerol. Al was beside me cooling my face and wiping my mouth after I vomited and just trying to comfort me. I had approximately five contractions when I got a sudden urge to push. I told Al I had to push, but I was having difficulty with the breathing technique where you blow and push. He instructed me on how to blow out properly and then called the nurse. I remember feeling scared because I didn't think I should be having this pushing urge and was afraid I would not be dilated enough.

At 1:05 a.m., the nurse came in and checked to see how far I was dilated. She told me I could push. She held one knee while Al held the other knee against my chest. She instructed me on how to push, although I had a good idea from the classes. I blew the first push because instead of holding my breath and pushing, I blew out. I quickly got the hang of pushing and I thought it was a great relief to the labor pains. In fact, I could hardly wait for my next contractions so I could push some more. After about four pushing contractions, Al went to get changed into delivery room clothing (Remember, this is 1983). The nurse told me I would be given the epidural when they could see the baby's head. Both Al and I asked her if I would need it at this point and she said that it was my first baby and it might hurt me. I felt confused because I had Al on one side saying to me that I shouldn't have one because I was pushing now, and on the other side the nurses saying it's your first baby. I asked the nurse what it would feel like because the pushing felt great but she wouldn't comment.

They started to wheel me to the delivery room. I was still undecided about the epidural. I found it very difficult to make any decisions when I wanted to push so badly. I remembered from conversations in our Lamaze classes that an epidural shouldn't be given after you are in transition.

When I got to the delivery room, I finally decided I was not going to have the epidural. A minute later a nurse came in and told me "The doctor wants you to have an epidural." Both Al and I told her I didn't want one. The doctor entered the room and said to me, "I want you to have an epidural." I started to tell him NO, when I had another contraction. Al and the doctor argued back and forth while I was pushing like mad. He wanted to know what Al had against an epidural, and Al told him that it was too late because you could see about 2 inches of the baby's head. He said that was not a good reason. At this point my contraction had finished and I told him I didn't want one because it was too late.

He said, in a big huff, "Okay if that is what you want," and he threw up his hands. He went and sat down at the end of the delivery table and tapped his scissors very impatiently. Meanwhile, I had my left leg strapped in the stirrup and a nurse was trying to adjust the other one but it kept falling down. Al was annoyed at this point and he made a comment about these stirrups must have been designed by a doctor and not an engineer. The doctor gave him a dirty look. I didn't care what was happening because all I wanted to do was push. The doctor gave me a local anesthetic. The part that hurt when pushing the baby out was when the shoulders came through and it was only for a couple of seconds. I was given a small episiotomy, but I wonder if I could have gotten away without one.

Ryan Benjamin was born on November 23, 1983 at 1:58 a.m., weighing 8 lbs. 1.5 oz. He first cried when placed on my tummy; at the same time he urinated on me. He looked healthy and beautiful with nice chubby cheeks. Both Al and I were ecstatic. I wanted so badly to hold him but the nurse took him to do the Apgar score (he scored 9) and put the silver nitrate drops in his eyes. They cleaned him up a bit and put him on a heated bed. They brought him over so I could see and touch him. After the doctor finished cleaning me up, I was transferred to another bed and finally they let me hold him. I held him for a few minutes and then they let Al hold him. After about 5 to 10 minutes they took him to the nursery, and Al and I went to the recovery room where we discussed how great the birth was and how useful the classes were, how bad mannered the doctor was, how beautiful and healthy looking Ryan was and what a relief that everything turned out so perfectly.

The nurses congratulated us on what a good job we did, what a good coach Al was. When I was on the delivery table it was Al who was coaching me with the pushing. The nurses stepped aside when they saw that Al I knew what we were doing. I am very thankful that Al was there for the labor and the birth. He was so helpful and

I am especially thankful that he talked me out of having the epidural because I would have had one and regretted it later. I would have also missed out in the great sensation of pushing the baby out.

For the first two days following the birth I had approximately eight hours sleep and felt so excited and full of energy. On the second day, the pediatrician told me Ryan was healthy, but slightly jaundiced. He would be doing more tests and there was nothing to worry about. On the third day he told me Ryan's jaundice was higher and he would have to go under the phototherapy lights. I knew it was not serious and there was nothing to worry about, but I think all the excitement, lack of sleep, and post-partum blues caught up with me and I started to cry my heart out. I had to go to a bath demonstration, so I got myself under control. When I came back to my hospital room I started to cry again. One of the nursery nurses came in to tell me about the jaundice and where he would be. She saw I was upset so she talked to me about what causes a baby to be jaundice, she also talked to me about breastfeeding and postpartum blues. I found the nurses to be very helpful.

Ryan and I were in the hospital for one week, which gave me a bit of time to find out more about bathing, diapering, and feeding him. Physically, I felt much better than I would have if we had been released when my doctor said I could go home (3 days after birth).

Both Al and I thought our Lamaze pre-natal classes prepared us very well for the birth. I used all the breathing techniques and found them helpful. We thought all the material discussed in the classes were necessary. We thought the classes were so good that we would be back for a refresher for our second child.

The Sweetest Thing

by Lisa Doran

For it was you who formed my inward parts;
You knit me together in my mother's womb.

I praise you, for I am fearfully
And wonderfully made.
Wonderful are your works;
That I know very well.

Your eyes beheld my unformed substance.
In your book were written
All the days that were formed for me.
When none of them as yet existed
Psalm 139: 13-14, 16

Authors Note: *This story was written in 1994 by my 24-year-old self. I was tempted to re-write it and craft the language a bit more so that it satisfies my 42-year-old ears today. However, reading it now and hearing my young, naïve and inexperienced voice makes me so proud of myself and of my wonderful partner Tim. So it is not changed, not one word, from the story I scribbled in my journal about a month after our first child was born. I had been a birth doula at this point for three years and had decided, even though I had never attended one, to have a homebirth. As luck would have it this was just one short year after midwives were legislated in Ontario and I had easy access to homebirth and wonderful caring midwives. Our son Jacob today is 18 years old and a wonderful young man who enriches my life in the most incredible ways. Thank you Jacob for allowing me to share this story of the day my life changed forever.*

My first child, Jacob Gaelen Doran, arrived here at 11:36 p.m. on December 9, 1994. He is so beautiful that it would just break your heart – but then I am a little biased! I am still awestruck sometimes. I cannot describe how happy and fulfilled I feel with this little person in our lives. Tim is absolutely bursting too. They look so wonderful together. A father and his son. Tim is so gentle and patient and loving with Jacob. It is really beautiful and it brings tears to my eyes sometimes when I watch them together. We are so lucky.

I was nine days late and that kind of sucked because everyone kept telling me that since I had preterm labor at 25 weeks and was having very strong Braxton hicks since 34 weeks and because I was carrying this babe so low that I would probably be early. Wrong! I expected to deliver in mid November! Waiting really got to be trying at times, especially with some members of my very large and loving family calling every day to ask if the baby had come yet! Tim and I decided that with the next pregnancy we are going to tell everyone that our due date is two weeks later than it really is so that our families will leave us alone!! Jacob came when he was ready and not a second sooner.

The labor was a very positive experience for me and I feel really great about it. I lost my mucous plug at about 9:00 a.m. on Friday. My midwife, Jennifer, called at about 10:00 to remind me to book a biophysical ultrasound because that is policy with 14 days overdue for moms who are planning a home birth. I told Jennifer about the mucous plug, and she said in her knowing way that it could still be days, so not to get too excited. I was having cramping pains – like a bad period, but they still were not definable enough for me to call them anything different than the crampy pains that I had been having since September.

I took the homeopathic remedy Caulophyllum 200 CH hoping that this was the real thing. I watched the birth video "Special Delivery" while Tim had breakfast, and I snuck upstairs and used my breast pump to stimulate my nipples hoping for an oxytocin release and some real labor. I had read somewhere that women who stimulated their breasts 3 hours a day usually went into labor right on their due date so I decided to try it. However, I could not imagine how they managed 3 hours a day, so I decided to do a half hour with the breast pump whenever I felt like it during the day. I only needed to do it twice! I don't know if this was a factor or not, but it may have helped. Tim thought that it was pretty strange, but I was frustrated because I was so uncomfortable and I had tried just about every other non-invasive thing that I could think of, including acupuncture.

So I spent the day tidying up a bit; Tim went off to work. I watered my garden and cleaned up the back yard. It was raining and cold out so I didn't go for my usual afternoon walk. At about 2:00 p.m. I went for a nap and I woke up at 3:30 with stronger, more regular cramps, still nothing too severe, but regular. When the cramps got tough, I got down on all fours and breathed really nice and slowly. It helped. I also started to use some visualizations and affirmations. I called Tim's lab at McMaster University and asked him to come home, and I called Jennifer again. She wasn't too concerned that anything was imminent and said that she would call back by 6:00.

Tim got home at 5:15 or so (I had said not to rush) and we watched "The Simpsons" and then he went to the grocery store to get some stuff for a pasta supper. We hugged a lot and we were both excited because I knew that this was more than just cramps. I called mom and let her know what was happening. It was freezing rain here and the roads were miserable and I told her that she didn't need to come – but she said that she was coming anyway. A 6-hour drive braving black ice could not keep her away from the birth of her first grandchild.

I had a bath while Tim went to the store. Jennifer called and I told her that I was getting some more bloody mucous but that nothing had changed. Cramps were still only 10 minutes apart and not very strong at all. When they came I labored on all fours because no other position was comfortable. She said to relax and go to bed early, but to let her know when I thought I needed her and to give her a good hour because the roads were bad.

Tim started dinner, and we sat down together and snuggled up to watch "Star Trek," which was a nightly dinner time ritual for us. My labor changed quite suddenly. Tim called Jennifer at 6:45 or so and let her know that my contractions were coming very close together and lasting a minute. There were still not as strong as I thought they should be. They still didn't really hurt, they were more distracting, that's all. I kept telling myself to trust the process, to give in to the process, to just go with it. I breathed deeply and tried to relax. I used my visualizations and affirmations. Tim told me to imagine that I was a big peach and that my uterus was a peach pit. My uterus was supposed to be hard while the rest of me was soft. That imagery made me giggle but it worked remarkably well for me! I truly felt soft and juicy.

Jennifer arrived sometime between 7:30 and 8:00 and spent an hour setting up the bedroom. We called our doula, who was also a student midwife and was supposed to help Tim coach, but she had gone out for the evening, so we left a message. Tim ran around finishing supper, helping Jennifer set up and helping me cope with my labor. He was fabulous, very calming and centering and encouraging.

Jennifer checked me at 9:00 and I was 5 centimeters dilated stretching to 6 during a contraction. Not bad for 4 hours! My doula and the back-up midwife arrived. It was snowing now. Everyone commented on the weather. How awful it was outside, how cold and bitter and how dangerous the roads were. How winter had just suddenly arrived. I was thankful for my cozy and safe nest. Thankful that I didn't need to go anywhere or worry about anything except my labor and my baby.

I was still laboring kneeling at the couch and that felt good, but it was hard on my sore knees. I wanted another bath, so I had a warm candle-light bath, lying on my side in our tiny townhouse bathroom. Jennifer ladled water over me, and I felt absolutely wonderful. I fell asleep during contractions and started using vocalizations when I could feel them build inside of me. I liked how my voice sounded in that small room. The echo. The resonance. Tim took over ladling and encouraged me to use my voice. It was very relaxing and wonderful. Between contractions Tim and I talked a little about how things were going and I warned him that transition was coming up and that for some women it was a tough stage. I got out of the tub and put on a flannel nightie and went to bed.

I did need a lot of support during transition – everything got very intense then and I had a hard time giving up my control and focusing on relaxing. Tim was fabulous, very calming, centering, supportive, and encouraging. He had to work harder to keep me focused and centered but his constant reassuring presence helped. I was getting discouraged and cranky and feeling really mean. I couldn't seem to visualize as well as I had before and I had forgotten my affirmations. Tim was wonderful. He rubbed my back and encouraged me and was there for me the whole time. He was my rock that I clung to when I felt I was going to be swept away.

I started to feel a lot of pressure and I kind of wanted to give a little push. Jennifer told me not to and checked me again. I was 8 to 9 centimeters, but my waters hadn't broken yet, so she hooked them and they gushed all over the place. Transition only lasted about 45 minutes or so. I decided that I wanted another shower so we all went to the bathroom. I sat on the toilet and really felt a lot of pressure. I couldn't breathe through a contraction anymore. I wanted to push. My body started pushing for me – so we went back to the bedroom and I got on all fours on the bed. I wanted to push. Jennifer did another exam and I still had a lip of cervix so I had to pant pant blow through two contractions. The pushing urge was too strong. My midwives kept saying, "Don't push," and all I could say is, "I AM not!" The urge is completely involuntary. When Jennifer checked again my baby's head was past the cervix and I was allowed to push. Boy it felt wonderful to give in to that urge. It really was the most powerful and wild thing that I have ever felt.

I pushed for 11 minutes only and then Jacob was born. I was very surprised that he was a boy. I honestly expected a girl, but it didn't matter. He gave out a big wail and then turned his beautiful eyes on me. I was in heaven. I was in love. The whole thing, including my placenta, took less than 6 hours. I loved labor and birth. I loved holding my brand new son in my arms. There will never again be a time in my life when I will be as powerful, as beautiful or as filled with pure, wild instinct. I really felt a connection with the deeper rhythms of life that night.

Tim cut the cord and I was bleeding and torn from Jacob's shoulders coming out as quickly as they had. Tim held Jacob for almost an hour while they fixed me up. I needed oxytocin to stop the bleeding and two stitches for my laceration. Mom arrived, disappointed that she had missed the birth, but thrilled with Jacob. The midwives changed the sheets and washed me up a bit and then everyone left Tim and me alone for an hour with our son. It was really great. We had a beautiful hour together, loving each other. We had a glass of wine and I had something to eat. The birth party moved downstairs for pierogi, cabbage rolls, and our wedding cake that we had frozen 3 years ago. After that Jacob and I had a warm herbal healing bath, and then I put on a new nightie and we went back to bed. My sister Jeni arrived and my step dad Julian came upstairs – they were both thrilled. We called my other sister Becky in Hawaii and she cried. She was really happy for us.

The biggest thing I learned was how wise my body was. My body grew and nurtured Jacob for 9 months and then my body knew when it was time for Jacob to be born and my body completely did all of the work. It is strange. In labor you really have to kind of put your brain on hold because it isn't your brain that is running the show. You really have to give up control and just trust that your body has the wisdom to do its job.

Jacob weighed in at 8 lb, 7 oz and was 52 centimeters long. He was perfect at birth. Jennifer calls my birth "precipitous." I thought that it was one of the most powerful, wild, wonderful, and empowering things that I had ever felt and I was so thankful that we decided to do it at home, where we were left alone to do our own thing and where the process of birth and labor was respected and honored. The midwives treated Tim and me like we were the only two people on earth. It was a really wonderful experience for me. Having midwives was definitely the way to go. They took such good care of me. They visited us every day after the birth for a week to be sure that everything was going well and that we were both healthy and happy. The care has been wonderful. Midwives are really *care*givers in the full meaning of the word.

And the sweetest thing? Joyful Birth. Wild Mama, Strong Mama, Beautiful Mama. Gentle Daddy, Sweet Man, holding your son. An angel sent to live with us, love with us, and remind us to be forever filled with gratitude for each other and for our many blessings.

Remembering to Breathe!

by Elisa Bisgould-Menendian

I AM TRULY THANKFUL THAT ALL OF the births I have had the fortune of attending have been what I would consider to be joyful, or full of joy. To me, the definition of a joyful birth is one that invites peace, thankfulness, awareness, and, of course, joy, or the feeling of happiness and pleasure to the new family and to those sharing in the precious moment of welcoming a new human being to our shared planet.

I locked my car, thinking how fortunate I was to have found such a great parking spot. As I clumsily took my things from the car, shaking a bit with nerves, I breathed. I pushed the button for the intercom, I breathed. I stepped into the elevator, I breathed once again, and as the doors opened I took another deep cleansing breath thinking that now I was here for someone else, my "stuff" was not part of this. Knowing that my family would be fine because I had prepared for this, knowing that I would be fine because I too had prepared for this.

As the elevator door opened, I was greeted by dad and soon to be older sister with a feeling of joy, anticipation, and calm. This family was on its way to becoming a family of five. Midwives were sitting taking notes, chatting in a quiet hum. Mom was walking in the house, talking and taking contractions in stride. The eldest sister joined in the room with her purse and video game, while the youngest daughter breastfed, which of course assisted with encouraging the development of contractions.

I was in awe!

Was I needed? What was my role?

How could I help these people I barely knew?

I am still new at this.

They have invited me here, they are paying me!

How will I prove to them that I am worthy of their trust?

Everything seemed to be flowing so beautifully.

Would I be in the way?

But as time passed, I discovered that, of course, I was needed, as well as welcomed and truly as part of the team that would be fully involved. As I slowly became settled and organized, mostly within my own head, I watched a beautiful dance unfold before me.

Children gave mom and dad big hugs and kisses before leaving. They also kissed mom's tummy with the knowledge that when they returned they would be big sisters to their new baby brother. It was so beautiful to watch the love this family had for one another. What truly touched me was the naturalness of it all.

Breastfeeding, contracting, chatting, hugging, kissing, walking, talking, cooking – truly joyful!

As a doula, I was prepared to step in to "help". I was waiting for my "big cue". Slowly I realized that there was not going to be a big cue. My role was to participate quietly, ask for, or go to retrieve a drink for mom, a pillow, try to do anything I could to increase mom's level of comfort, as she continued to breathe calmly and effectively through each contraction.

She maintained a tranquility that was lovely to watch and a beauty to marvel at. Each contraction came and then went away. We waited and prepared for the next one. We worked together, the midwives, dad, and I, to support mom through each moment. Each contraction she experienced included a deep breath and quiet rhythmic breathing until at last, the contraction ended and was washed away with a cleansing breath, … by all of us!

Throughout labor, I found myself spending much time squeezing mom's hips, reminding her to breath, shaking out my wrists as the numbness set in, learning and listening to the experience the midwives were sharing with each other and with me, and, somewhere in the back of my head, reminding myself, that I needed to remember to breath too.

As mom was encouraged to push past the pain, I was reenergized and felt an overwhelming sense of hope and power. There is a power in being a doula, it is the power that comes from knowing that a mom can do it, from knowing that her partner is mighty in his/her role and from knowing that when we all work together, to support and respect each other, an incredible event will occur … and it will be joyful!

As I encouraged and reminded … and breathed, a baby is born! I was excited!

He emerged from his mom and was then placed immediately onto her chest. No one had yet confirmed if baby was a boy or a girl, everyone was just so excited that baby had arrived!

Delivery of the placenta, another miracle of life came soon after. As the midwife examined its perfection, the tree of life was pointed out and I was amazed. What a beautifully wondrous event I had just witnessed and participated in! I felt so blessed and fortunate to have been given the highest honor. I was there to witness the miracle of life. I was there to share in the joy.

As I quietly excused myself, not wanting to disrupt the flow and peace that had now entered the space, I took a moment to stand back and breathe while taking in as much as I could. I wanted to remember this. I wanted to take a picture in my head. I knew that a regular photo would not possibly capture what was happening in this home.

I watched as grandma and dad took turns holding and celebrating this new child, welcoming him to the family, I couldn't help but smile, feeling encouraged about the power of new life and the hope this tiny little boy symbolized. Big sisters would arrive home later to meet their new brother and new friend. I couldn't help but smile, feeling encouraged about the power of new life and the hope this tiny little boy symbolized.

A family had grown.
A new baby was here.
Everything was perfect. Everyone was full of joy!
(Including me!)
…now breathe!

Little Dove

by Joanne Raines

WHEN I WAS EXPECTING MY SECOND child, I purchased a sweet little story book entitled *The Day You Were Born*. While we looked forward to another baby, our first child loved that little book and after each reading, he'd want to hear the story of the day he was born. On our evening walks home from daycare, we'd pass a fountain and each evening he'd throw a penny in and wish for a baby brother. His wish came true and we often share the story of the pennies. Our birth stories are important not only to us as parents, but also to our children.

This is Little Dove's birth story:

It was a misty, Monday, November morning as we walked peacefully through the woods in the conservation area behind their home. The rain had changed to mist and the fog had set in just as I joined them on the morning of their beautiful birth. A few months earlier I'd met my clients and one very gracious Grandma, who was here from Latin America to offer support and share in the joy of their pregnancy and birth of the baby who would be welcomed into their family. Right away we were comfortable with each other. Their hope was for a home birth surrounded in love with things special to them. They were cared for by two midwives from a practice a little ways away – one very experienced and one fairly new. At each of our prenatal meetings, these expecting parents shared their thoughts and wishes as we prepared for the birth of their first born – a girl. Over the next while, they began to gather and nest, arranging everything for her arrival. They, as well as family members abroad, were looking forward to meeting this baby girl.

So on that misty November morning when my clients called to let me know it was their birth time, I was excited for them. Being a doula is not what I do, it's who I am. A path that began many years ago. With each call to birth, I anticipate the unfolding of another family's story where my role is only to offer guidance and encouragement. I believe in birth and I believe in them.

I learned that Mom had been laboring through the night, that midwives had been by and that all was well. The couple had slept and were now awakened with labor well underway, and they felt it was time for me to join them. When I arrived, Momma was breathing calmly and vocally. With each outbreath, she toned the vowels: Aaa – Eee – Iii – Ooo – Uuu. A calm, relaxed momentum filled the room. Her hands were open and relaxed – no tension – she called them frog hands.

Momma decided she'd like to take a walk in the woods and allow gravity to help in bringing her baby down. Off we went through the fog (cell phone & ID in pockets) and she led our way to the conservation area. With each surge, we'd stop and breathe through, together. Soon we came to beautiful wooded spot. She told me it was a place that she, Dad and Grandma enjoyed so much. That it was her favorite place because it reminded her of where hobbits might live. A few more steps, a few more breaths and we'd move on. A bit further along we arrived at a little bridge – stop – breathe – listen to the water trickling underneath – and walk on. This Momma talked about the future; of her and Dad walking here, with their baby. The serenity of nature was a beautiful and comforting place for her to labor.

When we arrived back at their home, Momma ate a little lunch and practiced yoga while Dad prepared food for Grandma, himself, and me. He was excited about this baby girl's arrival and trying hard to keep busy. It was so sweet to share in his excitement. As her surges became stronger and closer together, Momma continued to rely on her relaxed breathing rhythm and rituals with Dad by her side. She was tired, but able to close her eyes and rest between contractions, taking advantage of the little breaks to rejuvenate. The midwives were called to let them know that baby's time was getting closer. Upstairs I filled the tub, so the warm water would soothe her when she stepped in. Dad brought cold drinks, an icepack, and offered loving words of encouragement.

When the midwives arrived, one set up while the other moved closer to Momma. She checked and shared that baby would be born soon. Momma was doing so well and was encouraged by knowing that she would soon have her baby in her arms. Earlier, Momma and Dad had swayed together in the dance of birth. Now he placed on her neck an amulet that had been passed down through generations and got down close to her face, encouraging her with quiet, loving talk. The bedroom was calm, strings of white lights lit the room, and Bach's soft cello music was playing. Momma moved to the bed.

One more surge. A wee head with lots of dark hair. One more surge. A perfect body with delicate, beautiful skin and she was placed skin-to-skin on Momma's chest. Momma and Dad were so happy as they shared her in wonder and I stepped away. Beethoven composed *Ode To Joy* and in joy the new parents welcomed their little one.

Grandma had waited patiently downstairs and now I let her know, "Todo es bien" (all is well). Soon it was time to go up and meet her first granddaughter! She gave thanks that Momma and baby were healthy. And she was so proud. When the baby's name was announced, I learned that it means "Little Dove." In tears of joy we all toasted her safe arrival.

Just a few short years later, I had the honor of joining this family once again and we welcomed their second child. During our talks, they shared with me that they continue to walk in those woods together. They told me that when they walk they recite to "Little Dove" the paths and places of labor and that she treasures the story of her birth.

Mary's Healing Birth

by Mona Mathews

MARY CONTACTED ME IN HER 38TH week of pregnancy. I am usually hired earlier than this, but I had the feeling she didn't want to think of what was ahead and now that she was possibly just two weeks away, she needed to get ready. She had two older children, daughters ages 10 and 12. This wasn't a planned pregnancy, she had an IUD in place since her last child was born. I met her at her OB's office. She told me she felt she needed to hire a doula this time.

She had a very traumatic birth experience with her first child. She labored for hours with little to no support. It was a long weekend, and the hospital was short staffed. She and her husband noticed that the baby's heart rate was very high on the fetal monitor and stayed high. Her husband alerted staff because they knew something was wrong. Their fears were brushed off, and it took forever for a doctor to attend to her. Eventually, a nurse came into the room and there was a lot of commotion, she was given an episiotomy and forceps were used to deliver the baby who was born limp and not crying. She was worked on for quite a while, and eventually took her first breath. After they came home, she did not develop like the other babies in their neighborhood, and then the seizures started. No one took any responsibility for what had happened to this child at her birth. They were immigrants to Canada and did not have the money to take legal action.

After a couple of years another child was born. Although Mom had a lot of fear, this baby was born after an epidural ... healthy. Mary suffered with postpartum depression for months, just as she had with her first daughter. She thought her childbearing years were over, but now at 40 she found herself carrying another baby. She was determined to have this child with no medical interventions, and in as natural a way as possible. As natural as one can have in a hospital with an OB.

That is why she hired me, and we formed a connection right away. I believed in her and understood why this was so important to her. I encouraged her to read *Spiritual Midwifery* by Ina May Gaskin, to drink plenty of water, to see her RMT, chiropractor, and naturopath. We practised the comfort measures I would incorporate during the birth. I massaged her hands and feet and we listened to relaxation CDs of nature sounds and crashing waves and read positive birth affirmations.

Mary no longer had faith in traditional medicine, but like many women in Ontario the midwives in her area could not take her on; they were fully booked during the period of her due date. Two weeks since our initial introduction, at 40 weeks term, her OB started talking induction. Mary was determined and advocated well for herself. No, she would not agree to an induction. Then she reached 41 weeks. This time, after much more pressure, she again refused an induction, but did agree to go to the hospital for a non stress test and biophysical profile. Anyone who has undergone these tests quickly learns that going to the hospital, finding a place to park, going to the ultrasound department and then to the maternity department and waiting your turn takes up most of a morning. Mary felt like she was buying herself some time.

Her first tests were on a Monday. "Baby looks great and is healthy. Come back on Wednesday for the same test." She went back on Wednesday, with the same results. "Baby looks good, but is large. You should agree to the induction." Mary said no. She went back on Thursday, same results. "All is well, but won't she consent to an induction?" No. She went back on Friday. Baby is still doing well. What comes after Friday? The weekend! No tests will be done on the weekend. Wonderful! Maybe she will relax enough to go into labor on the weekend. Father's Day is Sunday. Wouldn't that be a wonderful Father's Day?

Saturday morning she called me. After speaking to her almost every day for the past week and offering encouraging words, telling her how incredibly strong she is to stand up for her rights even though she was being urged daily to submit to an induction … to say that she has decided to ask for a c-section! What? I couldn't believe my ears. "A c-section? Mary you do not want a c-section." She was so afraid that she would have to be induced that she would rather consent to a c-section. I calmed her fears and said "let's see what tomorrow brings." Wouldn't you know it, she called me at 8:30 Sunday morning. She was in labor. Her surges were coming quite regularly, about 6 minutes apart. Looks like I would be attending a birth today, I thought to myself. It didn't matter what family plans we had of our own that weekend, I was so excited for her.

An hour later, she called me again and we decided to meet together at the hospital. She was moved straight to a room as her surges were now coming every 3 minutes and she was struggling to get through them. We had a lovely nurse, Carol, who examined her and declared her to be 7 centimeters dilated. Mary's two older female children were shown where they could wait in the family waiting room. Carol was a great source of support and suggested that Mary go into the jetted tub. Mary breathed very deeply through her surges, and after an hour Mary's girls were brought in to see their Mom and were told the baby would be here very soon. Mary came out of the tub to be checked and was 9 centimeters dilated.

Carol called her "a house on fire" because she was moving so fast. I brought in the squat bar and very quickly Mary moved onto the bed. First, she stood and held the bar, and then with each surge she squatted and started to push. I was in awe of her. She was standing on the bed holding the squat bar, Carol and I on each side of her, and her husband Don encouraging her all the way. Now I had heard other doulas talk about "roaring Mamas," but I had never really witnessed it until this day. This Mom roared her baby into the world. She asked, "Do I have to wait for the doctor?" Carol replied, "Only if you want to."

The doctor did make it in time and was very gentle and respectful of the way Mary wanted to birth. He allowed her the time for her perineum to stretch and baby eased his way out. I don't always watch babies being born ... much of the time I am at Mom's head, but Mary was doing such an amazing job she didn't need my guidance, she didn't need anyone's guidance, she just eased her son into the world very slowly. She willed him into the world. I loved seeing first his head, and then the rotation of his shoulders ... he reminded me of an astronaut, almost weightless and effortlessly moving into the world.

The doctor was respectfully waiting for the cord to stop pulsing before clamping and I cut the cord, as Dad declined. Baby David was beautiful ... all 10 pounds of him with a shock of strawberry blond hair! Mom didn't even need a stitch. Mary was so happy and soon David was introduced to his very adoring older sisters. Dad was beaming as he held his son. This is a picture I carry in my head ... the happy family around Mom's bed. A Father's Day I will always remember.

Mindful Birth, Joyful Birth

by Robin Gray-Reed

WHAT IS IT ABOUT BIRTH THAT GIVES it the capacity for bringing so much joy? I have often wondered this to myself on my journey as a doula, lactation consultant, and (most recently) nurse-midwifery student. At first, I was under the impression that birth was most joyful when it went smoothly, following the path that we most hoped it would take. I remember going home after attending births early on in my career as a doula thinking, "Well, that was a nice one, but it would have been better if ..." and listing to myself the bullet points on the mom's birth plan that she wasn't able to have. I'd go home and look at the pictures I took during the birth, seeing the overjoyed expressions on the faces of my clients as they met their baby for the first time, and wonder how I could have made it even better.

Maybe I could have done more to help her get through labor without an epidural, I remember thinking one time, after a client of mine with a posterior baby opted for anesthesia after hours of diligently working to turn her baby. In the photos I have just after she pushed out her baby and pulled her up onto her own chest with her own hands, she is glowing with such a profound joy. She had no complaints about her birth experience when I spoke with her afterward. Yet in my perfectionism, I wanted her to have gotten everything she had originally asked for.

I had (and still have) a lot to learn about supporting families through birth. First, that neither their birth experience nor the outcome was about me. My best efforts to help a mother have a natural labor might find themselves face-to-face with some facet of the mother's or baby's anatomy or physiology that truly necessitated an intervention. I have come to see that my biggest gift to the families I serve is the quality of my presence with them during one of the most intense and life-changing experiences they will ever have. Taking my ego out of the equation and putting my heart in its place has been a hard but beautiful lesson to learn, and has increased my own joy at attending births. When my focus is not on perfecting their experience for them, I am freed to be fully present with them in that experience.

I realize this may be a controversial assertion to make, but I don't think it is the outcome of a birth (or any other experience in our lives) that makes it joyous. Rather, I believe that true joy comes from approaching any circumstance with the willingness to let it be what it is, whatever it is, and to be fully present with that reality in that moment without anxiously scrambling to make it be different. This approach, grounded in mindfulness, does not mean failing to take action if action is warranted; on the contrary, being mindful allows us to act with a clear head, unclouded by panic. Making the commitment to being open to whatever unfolds, moment by moment, has taken me on a journey that has changed my life and brought me greater joy than I ever knew possible.

It took me 40 births to learn that "a good birth" wasn't about natural versus medicated or vaginal versus cesarean. I somehow made it that long before any of my clients needed a cesarean, and I would be lying if I didn't give myself some of the credit for my statistics. I had long had mixed feelings about my own birth (by cesarean), thinking that my mom might have had a successful VBAC with me if she had just been willing to try. Her OB offered her the option, late into her pregnancy, but she was already mentally prepared for another surgical birth and felt afraid of the unknowns of labor.

I was excited when the phone rang very early one morning. It was my fortieth client, who had been laboring all night and was ready for me to come over. I remember slow-dancing through her kitchen with her during contractions as the sun rose up over the mountains and feeling the most delicious sense of loving my life's work. I knew at that moment that I was exactly where I was supposed to be, and I was eager to welcome this baby into the world, playing it out in my head how I expected her labor and birth to go (following the birth plan, and with minimal interventions, of course).

Fast forward a day and a half. I had that same sense of joy and purpose as I sat with my client and her husband in the operating room and witnessed their daughter's cesarean birth. When that baby emerged from my client's body, I knew beyond any shadow of doubt that she had given birth just as rightfully as any woman ever had. I was also flooded with a profound sense of gratitude for what my own mother went through to bring me into the world. Any sense that surgical births were somehow less valid a way to birth were gone after supporting my client through labor, seeing her courage in meeting each contraction, witnessing the love her husband showed as they worked together to bring their baby into the world. After the decision had been made to perform a cesarean section, but before we went back to the operating room, my client looked at me and said, "I don't regret any of this. All of these hours I spent in labor, I felt so supported and loved, and I found my own power as a woman to give birth to my baby. I wouldn't change a thing about this experience."

Hearing her say that forever changed the way I practice as a doula, as well as the way I live my life outside of offering birth support. Sometimes it isn't in getting what we think we most want that we find ourselves most overjoyed. Sometimes, in the process of getting everything we think we'd most rather avoid, and in keeping our hearts open to the process of life anyway, we make room for a deeper joy that nothing can ever take away.

Fast and Fabulous

by Michelle Sliva

MY FIRST BIRTH EXPERIENCE WAS the most exhilarating experience of my life. For over 40 weeks of my pregnancy, I was terrified of labor simply because I am scared of pain. I thought for sure I would require pain management, but I surprised myself by going completely natural and I owe it all to my amazing birthing team of my midwives, doula, and best friend. My labor was a positive experience, and a happy memory I will cherish forever.

I knew I wanted a doula when my best friend had one at her birth. I was fortunate enough to watch the early stages of her labor and saw how vital the doula was in keeping my friend focused and in control. Right in front of my eyes, my friend would calmly go through each contraction with the doula coaching her through it.

I couldn't believe it! Where was the screaming, the cursing at the husband, and dramatic flailing of arms like in the movies? I didn't know it at that point, but that changed everything I knew about childbirth. When I became pregnant, I contacted my doula and loved her chirpy and warm personality. I immediately was drawn to her and knew she would be a great support person during my labor. After delivering five children of her own, running hypno-birthing classes, and years of being a doula, I knew she had the experience and knowledge. I felt relaxed with her and knew that her words and presence will help me have as calm a labor as possible. I didn't have a birth plan – I wanted to have an open mind so I wouldn't be disappointed. I wanted to find my inner strength to endure the contractions with control like my best friend. I remember when we left, I was telling my husband how lucky we were to snag her on our due date. My husband was very honest and said he was relieved to know that a professional would help me through labor and he could focus on supporting me in his own way.

On my due date, I would call my doula to complain why my baby was taking so long! I felt like a ticking time bomb and the daily cramping, and strong Braxton Hicks contractions were very confusing. I had no idea when I was going to "pop" and, emotionally, I wasn't sure I was ready to hold an actual baby in my arms. I would call my doula several times a day sharing my fears, apprehension, and frustrations and she was always so supportive and empathetic. She mentioned something that rang true at the moment: "Maybe labor can be stalled because a woman is emotionally not ready to go through labor and actually have a baby. Maybe you need to allow yourself to accept that, and find ways to distract yourself through the days so that your mind isn't consumed about labor."

So off I went doing small little tasks to distract myself. I baked, I went out to run small errands, I even did a maternity photo shoot! Finally, I was in a place where I was ready to conquer labor and hold my baby. I didn't know what I was getting myself into, but I knew I was ready and just as my doula prophesied, my actual labor began just days later!

My birth date started like any other day before that. I woke up with painful cramping scattered all over the place. But what was different about this cramping was that it wouldn't go away after walking around. I didn't know it at the time, but those were early contractions! I text messaged my doula complaining of the cramping, and she had a feeling that tonight would be "the night." She said she would keep her cell phone in front of her while teaching her HypnoBirthing class that evening. I told her that she could probably teach her entire class no problem and not worry about me at all! In the evening the cramping got stronger so I paged my midwife. She told me to have a bath and nap and then page several hours later to see where I would progress. I prepared a funny movie to watch on my laptop and within minutes I got my very first "real contraction!" I couldn't believe how much it hurt and how I felt my insides were squeezing and contracting as hard as possible. They were lasting about a minute and were roughly 4 to 5 minutes apart already! I was nervous and scared and immediately told the doula, midwife, and husband to come home right away! I called my best friend who lives 5 minutes away to say that this "was it" and she was over immediately to help me with the contractions before everyone else could come. She set the stage for my labor by helping me stay quiet and calm and focused. I bounced on the yoga ball, bouncing through each contraction, and I closed my eyes to find the strength and control through the pain. It hurt like nothing I ever felt, but I knew it was what my cervix needed to do in order to push out my baby.

About an hour later, the whole team arrived and I was already – 5 centimeters dilated. My midwife made me climb a flight of stairs to help move the baby down and eat a banana for energy! Through each contraction, I couldn't believe I was able to breathe through it and deal with the pain. My doula was there each step of the way, quietly supporting me in order to help me stay in control. After laboring for about an hour at home, I intuitively decided it was time to go to the hospital. Everyone started to pack up and prepare immediately. When we parked, it seemed that the hospital doors were 100 miles away! I wanted to walk in order to help move the baby down. I remember that evening was cold and windy, but I didn't really feel it since I was focused on the contractions. Apparently, the hospital lobby was packed with people, but I didn't notice. I was in my own world with the doula trying to find the strength to deal with each contraction with focus and control.

After the 45-minute trek to the hospital room, I was already 8 centimeters dilated. My midwife prepared me by telling me that I was in transition and my body would take over. The contractions were really intense now so I climbed on the bed and leaned on the bed frame so that I was upright. It felt most "comfortable" and I knew it would help bring my baby down. My doula would lock her eyes into mine with each contraction and it was like she took hold of my emotions. I was scared, I wanted to scream, and I remember saying, "I am done. I really can't do this." The doula supported me by saying I really can do this even though I doubted myself. She held my hand, looked into my eyes and gave explicit instructions on how to push and bear down with each contraction.

I trusted her completely. I was no longer scared but rejuvenated because I knew she would give me the support and instructions I needed to see my baby. During the next several pushes, I heard only my doula's voice and the rest of the world faded away. While groaning through the most intense pain of my life, I allowed each contraction to take over my body. It was such an overwhelming and terrifying feeling, but I trusted my doula. I probably would have seized up and fought against the contraction due to the pain if it wasn't for her coaching. I pushed and pushed and I remember worrying that my baby would come flying out since the sensation was so strong! She assured me everything would be fine, and I continued to push.

Moments later, my beautiful boy was born weighing in at a whopping 9 pounds 13 ounces! With only a small first degree tear and a couple of hemorrhoids, I delivered a beautiful little boy completely naturally in just over four hours. I remember holding him in my arms that first night and barely sleeping. All I could do was marvel at this beautiful little person I brought into the world. My labor was beyond anything I ever imagined. I was so lucky to have an uncomplicated and fast labor with such a great team. My doula was my emotional rock keeping me in control when I doubted myself. I owe so much to my doula. Because of her, I was able to give my son a medication-free birth and a calm delivery with a calm and happy mother.

♀ Birth to Me

by Millennia (Millie) Lytle

I was inspired to follow through.
I had watched my mother pregnant,
had babysat infants at 14 years old.
had moved into nanny at 18 for an 8 day old baby,
and remained in the house throughout the next pregnancy and birth.

I wanted to have my own so I started attending, I've realized
But little did I know that I would become
addicted to watching you be born.
Slow head, fast body.
Blue to pink.
Silent to crying.
Everyone watching
you are here.

Tears of joy and pride
Ultimate suspense

Empowered Birthing

by Jennifer Papaconstantinou

"WE'LL SEE. I'LL DETERMINE THAT," said the obstetrician. This was in response to our conversation of giving birth naturally – vaginally. As I left his office, I knew I would not be returning. This was touted as the best and newest hospital around, how could they be so close-minded?

I was 8 weeks pregnant with my second child, which left me confused and fearful. I knew I didn't want to relive the experience I had with my first. Options were what I was searching for...

Five years ago, my husband and I were young, newly married, and expecting. We did everything an expecting couple was to do: ultrasounds, doctors' visits, birthing classes at the hospital, read relevant books, organized the nursery, you name it.... I had pre-arranged the use of the new "Birthing Room" at the hospital where my doctor was Head of Obstetrics. This room was a new facility where laboring mothers could give birth peacefully, opposed to laboring in a room with two other ladies and their families. Looking back, it was anything but natural.

One evening, in birthing class, all the ladies had brought in their ultrasound pictures, except me; I didn't have one! A woman I had made friends with in class just so happened to work at an ultra-sound clinic and she offered a picture of the unborn baby growing within. While in the appointment, it was discovered that my baby was breech presentation at eight months. Now I knew why I couldn't breathe, and when the baby kicked I felt it low ... really low!

At my next appointment with my OB, I relayed the breech information to him, and much to my surprise, he told me that I had no clue what I was talking about. He stated that the ultrasound technician was wrong; he did not receive results from the clinic since it was simply a picture I went in for. Of course, he was the professional, so I never thought to challenge him – besides, I had never been pregnant before and he was the expert; so home I went without another thought about it all.

Early one morning soon after that appointment, my water broke, and off to the hospital we went, bags in hand and both of us feeling scared, not knowing what to expect. Imagine our surprise and shock when MY physician was not there. This had not been discussed with us – the probability of our physician not actually attending the birth – apparently this was the normal procedure for hospitals. Now we no longer were allowed to use the birthing room because my baby was breech! The automatic procedure for breech presentation was a cesarean section surgery! We were shocked and faced with big decisions; I was not consenting to surgery and was determined to deliver a breech child. Why not? I was delivered breech.

After careful examination, the physician on duty informed us of a footling breech presentation – one foot folded up, the other already down. This changed everything, as a footling presentation results in automatic C-Section surgery, no question. In the end, C-Section it was, which is a whole story in and of itself. Recovery was long and hard, but in return, I had a beautiful, perfect, adorable baby girl!

Now, five years later, I was faced with the fear that I might undergo the same emotional, physical, and mental trauma. My options were expanded when a close friend relived her recent experience with midwifery and I was interested and curious. The timing couldn't have been more perfect as the government was in the process of regulating Midwifery within Canada and the province of Ontario. The opportunity was very exciting and I accepted the referral and booked the appointment.

What a difference! In the past, I had made an appointment through the hospital reception, waited approximately an hour and visited with the OB for about 10 to 15 minutes. This time, I only waited for 10 minutes for a 1+ hour appointment. The joy! I was amazed and thankful for the support, knowledge and expertise these midwives offered. Even though this first appointment was in a clinic in a basement of a residence. At the second appointment, my midwife had received my medical records from the previous birth, which she voluntarily shared with me. It was at that time I discovered just how devious our medical system was – the medical record showed a normal breech presentation without mention of footling. As it turns out, I have been told, in the instance of a footling breech, Caesareans are a necessary surgery. Since I would not consent to the initial c-section for a breech birth; they had lied, scared, and coerced us into an unnecessary procedure. How wronged and violated I felt.

My husband and I decided to re-take birthing courses through a not-for-profit organization empowering expecting parents on labor, support, birthing, doula and breast-feeding choices. This time, we really did our homework, wrote our birth plan, and hired a doula to assist in labor.

It was in the last trimester that I finally convinced my husband to consider a homebirth. After careful consideration, research, discussion, and information overload, we made the difficult choice to switch. Much to our dismay, the decision was not supported by family and friends; it was actually met with animosity and anger! People were throwing out words like "neglectful" and "stupid." It was amazing to see how ignorant and powerless our society had become. Many believe that medicine is a necessary part of labor and delivery.

VBAC #1

I bought a blow-up pool from our local hardware store, new sheets, a home birth package, and the nursery was ready to go. Our daughter, Alexandra, now 5, was attending this birth so her education was also fundamental. The long-awaited day finally came and the pool was an unending source of comfort and pain management; however, our doula could not make the event as she was at my friend's labor and birth – how exciting to be in labor at the same time! Her absence didn't waiver my determination; I had my husband, my daughter, and my best friend, plus midwives. In the doula's absence, the midwives quietly told my husband that women who were planning a Vaginal Birth After Caesarean (VBAC) are on a "mission." This day I was on a mission, a mission to prove I could do the impossible. I knew the power of my own body and I didn't like the limiting verbiage of the medical community, nor their textbook cases that taught what couldn't be accomplished. I disliked their limiting beliefs. I was on a mission!

In labor, may baby's heart rate dropped. It was a cause for concern and they let me know the problem as well as the solution. Get him out or have an episiotomy. I pushed him out with every ounce of being I had left and then required some stitches afterward. Fourteen hours of labor brought forth a VBAC of a 7 lbs 14 oz baby boy. We named him Joshua. It was a monumental occasion for all attending.

VBAC #2

Two years and two months later I had been experiencing Braxton Hicks for over 2 weeks with many alarming episodes of false labor. It was early morning and I didn't want to bother anyone AGAIN, but decided that if I was up, my husband should be too. We were thinking that this was it, so a call to the midwives was made – and so was the bed. I went for a shower and 15 minutes later – it was all over! I came out of the shower, threw on a nightdress and felt the overwhelming urge to push. I delivered Andrew, a 9 lb baby boy, while his dad was calling 911. My daughter Alexandra, then 7, was grabbing towels and my poor best friend who had just walked in to help was holding my legs. Andrew made it before the ambulance could, and the midwives arrived about a half hour later! Birthing doesn't get any more natural than that – let's just say we walked around in shock for a couple of days post partum!

VBAC #3

Two years and two weeks later, at home, Claire was born peace-fully and naturally with our closest family and friends. After only 5 hours of labor, she came into a world of soft lights, smiling faces, and love – nothing like what we experienced at the hospital or the shocking birth two years earlier. Our two million dollar family was now complete.

It is my desire in sharing my birth stories to have women be inspired and empowered. My advice to expectant parents, mid-wives, and doulas is to let Mother Nature take her course. In the many years of being a mother of four and a Clinical Holistic Nutritionist, I have heard many birth stories, some beautiful and too many others, horrifying.

There is a time and a place for medical interventions and con-ventional wisdom can be useful in certain instances. The key to unlocking the power within lies in knowledge; knowledge is power and women are powerful and magnificent beings.

The Power of Trust in Birth

by Alicia Montgomery

DURING MY TIME AS A BIRTH DOULA, I've witnessed the power of emotional dystocia. When a woman experiences fear, anxiety, or other kinds of emotional stress in labor, catecholamine levels rise and can reduce circulation to the uterus and placenta, rendering contractions ineffective, thereby stalling labor. The ability of the female state of mind to have such a strong effect on the physical process of labor continues to amaze me. This story is a testament that the opposite of emotional dystocia exists. This is a beautiful story about the power of a woman's trust in her physical body and her intuitive knowing (and a little about how much this woman taught her doula).

Before I met Holly and Mike, I had been a doula for 20 births. I'd had a range of experiences that included medicated and un-medicated birth, home and hospital birth, doctor and midwife attended birth. And a range of Moms from 18 to 47 years old, first-time mothers and experienced mothers.

Warning bells went off during my first meeting with Holly and Mike when they told me they were confident they wanted natural birth, but they were becoming increasingly concerned about the ability of their obstetrician to help them with this. In his practice, episiotomy and forceps delivery were apparently not uncommon and he had told them as much. In their eighth month of pregnancy, they had decided they wanted some advice from a doula! Up until this point in my doula practice, I hadn't made any strong suggestions to people that they might want to switch care providers to achieve natural birth. While I had some experience, I was still feeling my way through area hospitals and providers.

I sat at Holly and Mike's dining table during our interview, and I remember Mike shaking his head and adamantly telling me that they did not want a birth with unnecessary interventions. He asked me what exactly they had to do to ensure the most undisturbed birth in a hospital environment. Both he and Holly stared at me waiting for an answer.

So I suggested a local Alternative Birthing Center located within a hospital. I described the queen-sized beds, jacuzzi tubs, supportive caring nurses, and the little to no intervention. They were sold on the idea right away – no hesitation. They contacted the head midwife and they switched care with only a few weeks to go in the pregnancy.

On our first prenatal visit we discussed their birth plan. We talked about pros and cons of interventions, and I left them with articles on those topics so they could review some of their options before they made their preferences final.

Since Holly and Mike had hired a doula and were committed strongly to a natural birth so late in pregnancy, I wasn't sure if they would be emotionally prepared for the possibilities labor would throw at them. So for our next visit I decided to focus heavily on emotional birthing preparation and physical expectations for natural labor.

We worked through a visualization in which I had Holly and Mike close their eyes and we discussed the word "journey" and its definition (an act or instance of traveling from one place to another, something suggesting travel or passage from one place to another). This word is often used to describe labor and birthing and I thought dissecting it would be helpful. I asked her to think more about its definition and why one would use it to describe birthing a baby. After about 15 to 20 minutes of me working through this with her, I asked her and Mike to open their eyes and draw their feelings with pastels on the subject.

My main goal here was to have them not only accept but also appreciate that labor could be long and could be hard work (just as embarking on a journey would be these things), but that was normal, healthy, and often transformative. We talked for some time about this exercise and Holly seemed to take away a lot from it.

After this discussion, we talked about pain in labor. I tried to normalize the possible intensities so labor would not surprise her. I remember distinctly Mike turning to her and saying, "Well, honey, I'm kind of worried about you tolerating the pain of labor. You know when you stub your toe you don't handle it well." !!!! He was being brutally honest. Here I was a little speechless as Holly turned to him calmly, put her hand on his knee, looked him in the eye, and said with a sweet even tone, "This is different. This is childbirth."

During our discussion about labor, I told Holly that based on what I had observed the most important tool she could bring with her on the day of her birth was not book knowledge, not her birth plan, but complete *trust* in her body and the birth process.

The day of Holly's labor came. She called me on the telephone to tell me her waters had broken, but she was not feeling contractions. She contacted the midwife on call, who advised her to stay home a few hours and then come in if contractions did not start on their own.

As a doula this honestly is not my favorite phone call to get. Even though I have confidence that women will eventually have healthy labors, a great majority of the time they are slow to start after a premature rupture of the membranes. I know that hospital practices have quite strict guidelines about how quickly a woman should deliver after a rupture because there is a risk of infection. I also know that the body rarely cares much about hospital policies.

The longer Holly's body went without labor the more likely she was to face hospital intervention to synthetically induce contractions. If this was what was meant to be for this birth, it would have to be in a standard hospital room, no jacuzzi, no queen beds ...

nothing Holly had been hoping for.

I gave some suggestions over the telephone and asked her to keep in close contact with me throughout the day and to call if she needed me to come. She waited it out at home for a while, but decided to go to the birthing center mid-morning with still no contractions.

We talked every couple of hours. The birthing center gave her some natural induction suggestions like walking and using a breast pump to bring on labor. But the hours went on. Between my suggestions and their suggestions things were just not happening. Can you imagine? The birthing process was not listening to our commands!

In the early evening, Holly asked me to come to the birthing center. At this time she'd been there almost all day. They were still giving her more time. Holly sounded very confident and content over the telephone. She simply was requesting my presence because she thought it might offer some more help. I was excited to be there physically and met them at the birthing center right away.

When I arrived, Holly and Mike were sitting near one another chatting. The lights were bright in the room. The birthing pump was out waiting for its next turn to kick-start Holly's labor. The energy in the room, while fairly calm, seemed also to be "out of ideas," if you will. The things that had been done up until that point to help this labor start were methodical and proven, but I knew that our bodies didn't always listen to instructions from our thinking brains.

At this point, Holly told me she had experienced a few painless contractions that were very spread apart. This had been going on much of the day. It seemed Holly needed change. It felt to me that she needed permission to focus on only her and the baby and not the methods of getting the baby to come out.

I asked her if she was willing to try some things with me. She was very happy to do something different. First, I softened the mood in the room. I shut the bright lights to a minimum dim. I sprinkled some lavender around the room to bring a sense of peace and calm. I turned on some soft Indian flute music for background noise.

I then asked Holly to climb onto the bed into a hands and knees position. I suggested she do some pelvic rocks to help her baby move into a more optimal position just in case that might be a problem. I told her I would be massaging the backs of her legs and her ankles and that I would be pressing the pressure points above her ankles to stimulate contractions periodically.

Most importantly, I stressed that there must be quiet in the room, that Mike could be right near her touching and supporting but that no one talk. I asked her to go deep inside to a place where she could communicate with herself and her baby, a place where she could allow her body to move forward with this birth. And that we would hold this space for her to do that.

Within 5 minutes Holly had a contraction. Five minutes later another contraction. Not a short painless contraction like earlier that day, but a long minute-long contraction! I listened to her breath in the dark, and I knew something had changed. I was quite surprised at how quickly things seemed to be picking up. I thought it might even be a fluke – that the labor might slow down in a few moments. But she kept contracting.

After about 20 minutes of hands and knees, I suggested she might like to walk for 15 to 20 minutes. Holly seemed excited to walk. I remember holding a discussion with the midwife while I watched her and Mike walk up and down the hall, stopping to hold on to the railing and contract every 5 minutes. Holly came back after 15 minutes or so and wanted to sit on the birthing ball for a while. I thought this was an excellent idea so I went back into her room and sat with her and her husband. And then such a beautiful thing happened.

As Holly was sitting on the birthing ball for a contraction, I noticed a slight shake to her knees, a sign to me that she was entering active labor. Her eyes were closed as two tears trickled quietly down her cheeks. I remember thinking, "She is overwhelmed with pain. It is much more than she expected." I had no physical reason to think this other than tears. She seemed to be peaceful before then. But I just assumed maybe she had been experiencing an internal struggle that I hadn't picked up on.

She opened her eyes and looked to me and her husband and said, "I'm not crying because I am upset. I'm crying because I'm so excited, I feel our baby coming."

I can tell you as this woman's doula – the doula of this first time mother who asked me what to do to achieve a natural healthy birth for her baby and then ran out and did it, a woman who showed calm and confidence to this point through what potentially could have sent her into worry and made her a mess – I never doubted her process or her emotional well-being for one more moment after that. By golly she was going to have a baby that day!

Holly asked for a vaginal check and she was 4 centimeters dilated – just beginning active labor, as we suspected. From there the nurses and midwife left us to do more of what we had been doing. But they were growing a bit more concerned. The clock was ticking after all and she had been there all day and was only beginning her active phase. The worry was that her labor could go on quite a bit longer, which would increase her risk of infection. Still they gave us a lot of space to birth undisturbed.

A few hours passed. By now Holly was in the big jacuzzi tub. The room was still quite dark. The mood was of absolute peace and hard work at the same time. Mike was in the tub behind her and she was faced toward me so I could offer support through soft words and eye contact.

I had realized in this birth, like many others, that my role was unique. Not all women need the same kind of support from a doula. Holly had an energy around her birthing space that was so strong and sensual, especially for a mother who had never experienced birth before or witnessed another woman in natural birth.

Her experience seemed very close to a sexual experience. I had a strong sense that it was private and internal for all three of us in the room. I knew that minimal "help" from me was needed. That it was my job to help her maintain the energy she had by offering sips of water, cool rag, encouraging words but not too many or too often, and a hand for her to hold.

Her body softly rocked in the tub. He hips swayed from side to side and around in a circle. Her voice came out in very soft, quiet, pleasurable sounding moans. Her eyes stayed closed sometimes and other times stayed fixated on my eyes (something today she says is the most vivid part of the process for her).

I sat in awe of her experience. I had heard about orgasmic birth.

I knew she was not having an orgasm, but she was experiencing something transformative and deep. I could tell her labor was progressing but only because of the slight changes in the way that she moved, the length of her noises, the slight sweat on her face, and what her eyes told me.

At one point a nurse stopped by and whispered in my ear, "Alicia, you might want to consider asking her to get out of the tub or trying something different. We need her to progress now." The nurse's assumption was that Holly was still at 4 centimeters because she was still smiling and calm. I turned to the nurse and said, "No, I think we've got this."

Very shortly after Holly was confirmed to be complete. She moved from the tub to pushing out her beautiful baby girl onto the bed. The midwife turned to her after the birth and said, "I knew the minute I met you and these long legs that you were going to do this Holly." I could tell Mary had the same intuitions Holly did about this birth.

At a postpartum visit, I commented to Holly about the sensuality of her birth. I asked her what she felt helped her achieve this experience. She turned to me and said, "Alicia, you told me to *trust* birth. That is all I did." It was as simple as that for her.

There was plenty of time during the 15 hours or so before Holly's contractions started that she could have lost faith in her body. She had to sit in the hospital most of the day hoping and waiting for contractions that weren't happening. But I don't believe for a moment she ever didn't trust that things would be just fine.

I knew trust was an important component to birth before Holly's experience. Her acknowledgment that trust was the primary force that saw her through her process cemented my belief. Birth is more an emotional process than it is a physical one. I don't say that lightly. Birth is quite a physical experience and physical preparation is important. But the physical often does not perform without the emotional.

A Birth Without Fear

by Vicki File

WHEN THEY WALKED OUT THE DOOR after our first consultation, I knew that I wanted them to include me in their birth. I turned to a colleague and said, "I *really* need to work with that couple."

There was something about them, an air of calm that just seemed to envelop them. They felt empowered by the philosophies of "HypnoBirthing" and the classes they had taken. They were in a different universe than my clients to date … they really knew what they wanted from their birth and their request from me was one thing: my presence. They wanted me to help protect the sanctity of their experience despite the boundaries within hospital walls, and to help bring things back on track if they started to go off course.

They knew one thing. They wanted a birth without fear. She believed in the power of her body, and her ability to bring her baby into the world, and he wholeheartedly believed she could do it. He already looked at her with such respect; I could only imagine how he would feel after watching her give birth to their child.

We met a couple of times before the big day, and the one wish that stood out in their plan was to be able to labor at home as long as possible. There was only one thing that would prevent that. She had tested positive for Group B Streptococcus (GBS), and hospital protocol indicated she would need to head in right away if her membranes ruptured.

As nature would have it, her water broke first, without a contraction in sight. This meant no labor at home. For some women, that would have been defeat, sending them downward into a spiral of doubt and disappointment. Not her. When they arrived at the hospital, I saw them coming across the parking lot in the dark. They were loaded down with pillows and bags galore. I didn't even notice that at first. All I could see were their smiles.

In the hours that followed, waiting for labor to begin, and throughout the early stage, she remained in good spirits. They talked and joked in spite of their sleeplessness and patiently persevered. I suggested all the natural methods I could think of in an attempt to get things to progress (aromatherapy, acupressure, nipple stimulation, positioning), and they eagerly tried it all. We were trying to beat the hospital clock and the pressures for intervention.

As active labor began, the atmosphere became more serene. She tuned into herself and listened to her HypnoBirthing exercises with deep concentration. He stroked her hands and smiled encouragingly. Soon, she needed me. I began to apply pressure to her sacrum and massage her lower back and hips while she leaned over a ball, or on the bed. The contractions strengthened and lasted longer, and she remained controlled. Not one word of complaint.

Hours passed, and the sun began to show signs of rising. She was side-lying in the bed while I rubbed her back and arms. He was taking a much-needed break and napping in the corner. I was watching her breathe through each contraction, so steady, so in-tune with her body, when I noticed she began to reach for the bedside table and grip with all her might. She had the inherent need to feel grounded; transition was upon us.

With the same calm and ease, she navigated her way through this stage. He sat in front and breathed along with her, keeping her focused while stroking her arms. I put a cold cloth on her forehead to help with hot flashes and nausea, and massaged her lower back and thighs to help with the shakiness. The sun finished rising and soon something felt different. With each new contraction I noticed her body moved a little differently, like she was beginning to bring the baby down.

"Are you feeling pressure?" I asked her.

"Pressure..." She whispered, vaguely panting. I watched patiently and with the next contraction she smiled, ever so slightly and breathed, *pressure!*

The nurse came in and I said quietly, "I think she might be ready to bring this baby out!" Sure enough, 10 centimeters dilated and baby descending, she was ready.

She asked for the birth bar and began to breathe her baby down, squatting on the bed. Positions changed a few times, as did techniques, but I will never forget this part of the experience. She wanted spontaneous pushing, she wanted to let her body take the lead. The nurse hadn't experienced this before and was a bit at odds with it. She asked me to coach, not understanding that this woman, this mother, didn't need to be coached. I stood by and encouraged her. I was transfixed by the look on her face. Never before have I seen a client "push" with that look. She was smiling. It wasn't a huge, crazy smile, but the subtle, confident, and strong smile of a woman about to lay eyes on her baby for the first time.

After some time passed, the doctor came in and suggested a more aggressive, directed form of pushing, but she held strong in her belief that her body could do it. At one point someone asked, "Are you doing okay?" and she exclaimed, "I love this!" With each push, she became more radiant, and the baby's head appeared and stayed in sight a little longer.

As the baby crowned and finally pushed through fully, she let out one big "ouch." It was the only expression of pain or discomfort in 12 long hours.

This brand new, wriggling baby was placed on mom's bare chest immediately, and I tried to absorb everything that was happening at once. Dad had tears pouring down his face, tears that could only have been full of joy and immense pride. Mom looked absolutely amazed by this perfect little being in her arms. Like no mother I have ever had the privilege to witness, she bathed her baby's vernix-covered face in tiny little kisses. She began talking and baby looked up with absolute recognition at the sound of her mother's voice. Overcome with feeling, I noticed tears streaming down my cheeks as well. I was honored to be there, to be part of this incredible, natural, emotional moment. Not only was a gorgeous baby girl born that day but a beautiful new family had formed.

When I left the hospital room, baby was having her first meal from mother's breast and Dad was proudly contacting friends and family to spread the news. It had been 36 hours since I had stepped out of my bed, but all I could think about was how wonderful it would be to do it all again.

Joy

by Lisa Caron

♀

IT WASN'T UNTIL I HAD BEEN A DOULA for many years that I realized I was truly *present* when attending women in labor. Being with a laboring woman is the easiest time for me to be right here, right now, in this moment. The seclusion allows all the multi-tasking thoughts to drop away. This gift of being present allows me to gather joyful memories as I think back over the hundreds of women and families I've attended in homes and hospitals. There are so many, and different memories come to me on different days.

❖ I recall the first birth I attended, untrained with only my own wonderful birth as knowledge. The young woman laboring on the same day I had 13 years prior. As I sat watching the sun rise reflect across the wall, it felt like I'd done this dozens of times before. Looking at all the tubes and wires, hearing all the clicks and beeps around the sleeping 18-year-old, I asked the nurse if there was anything I should be doing. Her reply was, "No, you're only here to hold her hand and tell her she's doing a good job." It took me many years before I could truly appreciate her overly simplified statement. As a new doula, I thought my job was to make everything perfect. Sitting and doing nothing was foreign to me, but it forced me to be present, to find my rhythm, to be more available to a laboring woman.

❖ I recall many women finding their rhythm in labor. One by rocking in a rocking chair; another woman found it helpful to lift and lower her arm repeatedly as she counted; and another sang beautifully.

❖ I recall a woman lying in bed spooning with her husband, her face clearly telling me she was well into labor. He moved away briefly and she reached out for him, purring, "I need you to hold me."

❖ I recall the peacefulness as I sat in a quiet dark room with a 16-year-old and her boyfriend as they slept together in her hospital bed before labor became active. I've watched with a smile as I see partners trying for all the world to keep their eyes open during labor, knowing how much they want to be there for their partners. I've cradled a sleeping two-year-old in my lap while her mother also slept next to us in a hospital bed.

❖ I recall a 15-year-old laboring in a big Jacuzzi with her girl-friends feeding her popsicles. Later, I watched her push her baby out while her calm and peaceful family doctor sat beside her on the bed, full of gentle encouragement. All the while almost a dozen friends and family, babies included, waited anxiously in her labor room on the other side of the curtain.

❖ I've watched a baby born in to his mama's bed, the same bed he was conceived in and the same bed I watched his brother and sister born on to.

❖ I recall trying to convince partners that couldn't comprehend how this baby could be coming so fast when the first one took two days. I've repeated a hypnotic forest scene over and over again to help a woman stay relaxed through an induced labor. It brings a smile to my face.

❖ I've kicked through the colorful fall leaves during a labor walk, and walked the purple labyrinth in the carpet of a downtown hospital.

❖ I recall kneeling next to a laboring woman at the side of her bed in the dark of night, as we had done twice before in the same room.

- ❖ I recall a woman shouting to her friend on the telephone moments after the birth of her second child: "I'm the queen of the world!" as she recounted her first unmedicated birth.
- ❖ I recall the absolute joy on a woman's face after the nurses and doctors worked so hard to help her accomplish a much desired vaginal birth despite extremely high blood pressure.

- ❖ Over the years I've learned how to wave a wet washcloth in the air to cool it so I don't have to leave the mother's side or reach away.
- ❖ I've learned how to give partners and family members errands and tasks to occupy their restlessness or help them stay awake.
- ❖ I've learned to help a husband crawl up on the bed and lay his head next to his wife's so together they could see their baby born onto her belly.
- ❖ I've learned to sit in silence and hold space, being present instead of filling the room with unnecessary chatter, and to sit in silence and listen while others find comfort in chattering unnecessarily.
- ❖ I've learned how to hug a policeman, bouncing off his Kevlar vest, in thanks for his last minute escort to the hospital in rush hour.

- ❖ I've witnessed women laying, standing, kneeling or floating in water as she pushes her baby into her own hands. I love to sit on the side of a tub waiting for the sound she makes in the middle of a contraction, "aaaah ... uh ... aaaah" when it's almost time.
- ❖ I've witnessed mothers who give in to the undeniable primal urge to lick their newborn. Or mothers who sniff and smell and kiss and can't get enough.
- ❖ I have witnessed a dad remove his shirt and stand next to the baby warmer, waiting patiently to hold his newly born against his bare chest.

✢ I have witnessed a father dance on the front lawn in celebration of their baby.

✢ I have witnessed the joy on a woman's face in a birthing pool as she first nestled her long-awaited son to her cheek.

As a doula, I have been invited to share memories that bring me joy; I have had the honor of witnessing intimate glimpses into the lives of families. These memories bring me joy and give me peace.

Welcome Baby James

by Nelia DeAmaral

AT OUR PRENATAL MEETING, WE talked about your various concerns. "What if I get the grouchy OB?" "What if they try to make me take drugs?" I could empathize with these concerns because sometimes there is too much meddling in the birth process, but at that moment, my doula "spidey sense" kicked in, and I said, "I just get a feeling that you will get the perfect OB and that the entire team will support you exactly in the way you want." I was right!!

The first call came in around 10:00 p.m. You told me that you were having somewhat mild contractions, but they were fairly regular. It was a courteous heads up to say things may or may not happen tonight. Within an hour, a call came from Gary. "She wants you to come now," he said, with some urgency in his voice. In about an hour, contractions went from somewhat mild to full on.

When I arrived around midnight, you were managing incredibly well! I could tell that things were moving quickly, but you worked at maintaining a calmness that is extremely rare when a woman is going through transition. We didn't know it was transition at the time, but we would soon find out exactly how far along you were.

We played HypnoBirthing CDs. You had a little snack and then hopped into the bath. Gary was always ready to anticipate your needs and provide loving encouragement. He was the ideal birth partner. Then, there was one really long contraction and a subtle little grunt at the end. We knew then that it was time to go!

Off we went to the hospital, running red lights (luckily Gary is a police officer, so I felt a little safe trailing behind him). It was a good thing. When you arrived, the nurses checked you and mayhem ensued. Gary motioned to me through the glass, trying to tell me that you were 9.75 centimeters dilated! I convinced the nurse to let me in where you were calmly laying on the bed while your body began to push your baby further down the birth canal.

Everyone moved quickly to get you into a room, and once we arrived, you began to move and breathe with the powerful urges to push. We tried several positions to make you as comfortable as possible. The doctor and nurses took a hands-off approach because they could see that you were doing extremely well without them! Everyone in the room supported you, offering drinks, cool towels, and words of encouragement. At no point, did you lose control. You were likely too busy to notice the admiring looks in the eyes of everyone around you. The doctor even said, "She came in at 10 centimeters? Incredible!" Most of the time, the obstetrician stood with her arms crossed smiling.

At one point, we brought in the mirror and you could reach down and feel baby's head. It was touching to see the awe in your face and the determination you had to birth your baby. After some incredible pushing, baby James crowned. The obstetrician delivered his head and shoulders then invited you to pull him out! You reached down, grabbed his adorable (and slippery!) body and put him on you. This moment touched me deeply as your doula. I felt the incredible strength and determination in you. You claimed your baby as the prize that you rightly earned. I felt myself well up with tears as I witnessed the power of you pulling your baby out. I have never seen an OB allow this, much less suggest it!

James was so strong and healthy. Within minutes, he wanted to nurse and he did, with almost no effort, and he stayed there for nearly an hour sucking and swallowing the colostrum that was already flowing freely.

Your birth is an inspiration to all women who know what is right for them and then go after it without allowing anyone to tell them that there is a "better" way. Welcome to motherhood!

A Wonderful Experience

by Heather Bradley

THIS IS THE STORY OF MY FIRST client. I had never been to a birth before, and I was very nervous about attending my first one. What a blessing it was that a good friend asked me to be her doula because I couldn't have thought of a better way to start my doula career. Her birth was amazing and empowering. Not just to other mothers, but to myself as a doula. Bearing witness to her birth gave me the perfect start to understanding just what our bodies are born to do.

My friend saw her due date come and go. For several days after, I had been waking to check my messages every few hours at night. I was worried I would sleep through the mom's labor alert ... and I almost did! If my youngest son hadn't woken up with a cough, I would have slept for a while longer. "Good morning! Wake up sleepy head!" was waiting for me when I checked my phone around 6:30 a.m. Reading those lines woke me up pretty fast! I knew that this mom was telling me to put on my doula shoes because it was time to get in gear. I sent her a message to see how she was doing, and she informed me that her contractions were coming every 4 minutes and lasting about 90 seconds.

I was *so* excited! In my doula training, I had learned that contractions 90 seconds long are a sure sign of labor progress and to head toward the hospital when they are 4 to 5 minutes apart and 60 seconds long for an hour. I threw on some clothes, quickly attended to my coughing son, and headed toward her house. I didn't make it very far though. The couple had decided it was time to head to the hospital and wanted me to meet them there.

It was raining out when I first left my house and pretty cloudy all the way to the hospital. I had never been to this hospital before, and I was afraid that I would miss it. I arrived at the hospital with little complication, even though I did take one wrong turn. The front desk wasn't expecting us yet, so I tried to wait patiently in the lobby. I got in touch with the dad, and we agreed that I would meet them out front and assist the mom while he parked the car. It felt like forever waiting, but I was soon to learn the value of patiently waiting...

The mom walked into the lobby with her headphones on and looked focused as she contracted. By this time, her contractions were coming about every 2 minutes. There were a couple of people in the lobby who looked concerned, so I made sure to give them a nice smile. I thought it might help them relax at the sight of a laboring woman, but looking back, perhaps I seemed really insensitive! My client was doing great though and walking and talking between contractions. After the dad finished up with admissions, they took the mom back to triage. Only one person is allowed to accompany the mom into triage, so I stayed in the lobby. This is where I learned the importance of being patient.

It was almost 2 hours before my client was moved to a room. I guess it was a busy day for the labor and delivery floor! I'm also sure that the lady at the front desk was tired of me asking whether the mom was still in triage. With the way she was moving along, I was worried that she was going to be delivering very soon ... and possibly without me. I would have been happy if she had a short labor, but I would be lying if I didn't admit I would have been disappointed to miss it. The dad finally came out to get me around 10:00 a.m. and told me that the mom was already at 7 centimeters dilation 90% effaced. The baby was at -1 station. That was such great news! She was sailing smoothly into the transition part of labor. When I got to the room, she was standing in the shower to get some relief from back pain. She still looked like she was able to stay calm and comfortable during the contractions. Her main complaint at this point (other than the back pain) was the obnoxious squeaking of the shower head. It was very distracting! The dad was holding the hose to help reduce the noise while I held her iPod close enough for her to hear. She had a great playlist of music prepared for every stage of birth, which seemed to be helping her relax. After a while, she decided to lie on her side in the tub. She wanted the water positioned on her back and the water to run in the tub. It really seemed to be helping her relax so we just followed her lead for support. She eventually asked for a cold rag for her face as it was flushing. This was also about the time she had a few hiccups. That was a very encouraging observation since I had learned flushing and hiccups are a sign of transition. I knew she was making good progress and started getting anxious to meet her baby. She was still very serene and able to stay focused through her contractions. The dad and I couldn't help but tell her what an awesome job she was doing!

She stayed like this for a long while until the midwife came to check her. Suddenly, it was very busy in the room. There was the midwife, a student doctor, and two nurses on top of the dad and I. The midwife wanted to get a saline lock started in case an IV was needed after birth and asked the mom to get out of the tub. A nurse tried to get the saline lock started while the mom was still in the tub but was having no luck, so the midwife said they could wait until the mom was in the bed to try any more. The problem was that my client did not want to get out of the tub. Well, rather she didn't think that she could. Her contractions were coming almost on top of each other so she was having a hard time moving. The dad and the midwife helped her out of the tub around 11:15. She had a good contraction on the way to the bed and leaned on the midwife through it. It was a bit funny because after the contraction, the mom apologized for getting the midwife wet.

Once in the bed, the midwife was able to check for progress in dilation. It was so exciting to hear that she was at 9.5 centimeters and the baby at 0 station! The mom was still listening to her music and singing in between contractions, which was very cool. There were a lot of people surrounding her at this point. One nurse was still working on her IV catheter, another nurse was monitoring the tocodynamometer and Doppler during contractions, the midwife and student doctor were getting the room prepped for baby's arrival, and other random people kept trying to come in. I was very pleasantly surprised to see that the hospital had such a good support system for laboring moms. The nurses were being very kind and courteous to the parents' wishes.

The mom was still feeling a lot of pain in her back, so I started to apply counter pressure with a hot pack. It seemed to be helping a little, but she was still pretty uncomfortable at this point. The nurse suggested that the mom may want to try getting on her hands and knees. The nurse, the dad, and I all helped the mom get turned over. By this time, she was having a hard time moving between contractions, and it took some teamwork to help her roll over. It definitely made it easier to get to her back to apply counter pressure. The dad and I rubbed her back and reminded her of what a great job she was doing.

Then, my client said she had completed that last half of a centimeter. Yes, she told us all when it happened! It was pretty amazing. By 11:45, she was feeling the urge to push … and then, there was the baby! The birthing team helped her roll over so that the baby could be put on her chest. She held him tight while the dad cut the umbilical cord. In fact, she didn't let anyone else hold that baby for a long while.

It was probably around 12:30 before the scale was brought in to weigh the baby. He had a good nursing before he was even weighed the first time. The mom kept saying he was so tiny, but he topped the scales at an impressive 8 lbs. 11 oz! The mom got up to use the bathroom and shower and it seemed like a great opportunity for a first bath for baby, too.

The room was starting to calm down finally. All of the staff had left and I felt like it was time to let the family bond. I was packing up to leave when the mom said she wanted to take a picture of me with the baby and her. It was a very happy moment for me. I felt so honored to be holding this baby, so new and fragile, at a time when I know his parents wanted nothing more than to hold onto him forever. It was the best present I could have gotten at the time.

I walked out of the hospital with my doula bag and ice cream (ordered for me by my clients) feeling a major buzz of happiness. It was such a wonderful experience for me. I may attend a thousand births after this, but this one will always have a special place in my heart.

The Many Faces of Joyful Birth

by Melissa Harley

WHAT IS "JOYFUL BIRTH?" THIS IS THE question I have been pondering ever since I heard the term. At first, I thought, sure, I could share some amazing, empowering birth stories where moms overcame obstacles to birth their babies in the way they desired. I could tell you of natural births where women still to this day surprise me by their strength, or I could tell you of the births where things went exactly according to plan and the mother, the new babe, and her family were cared for by their providers with grace, compassion, understanding, and true passion for their work. But after much reflection, I decided to go a bit deeper.

This year has been full of really amazing births in my doula world. I've had the beautiful home birth of a second time client who pushed out her 9 1/2 pound baby boy one beautiful fall morning. I've had the super-duper, speedy, heart-stopping, mom doesn't know if we're going to make it, births of not one, or even two, but six-yes six, babies! I've had the repeat clients, and I've had the new clients. I've had healthy boys and girls, and those who need a little more care. I've had dads who brought tears to my eyes by their involvement with their partners, and I've had those that preferred a different role. I've had the VBACs and the "text book" vaginal births. But in reflecting, to say that one was more joyful than another would be a misstatement, for sure.

What makes for a joyful birth? Is it if the birth goes as planned, if there are no complications, it is speedy (but not too speedy)? Perhaps it's because the family has those in attendance they want to be present. Or maybe it's more about the outcome of health of mom and baby. While all of those factors are relevant, I would say that they are not the causes for joy in birth.

Recently, I met this question face to face. I was at a conference, and surprisingly it was not a birth conference. For the first time in more than 16 conferences attended, this one was not for my profession or various leadership roles. This one was for me. I attended this particular conference in order to be inspired, renewed, and filled, and I left having experienced just that. I laughed and cried, reflecting on my many roles, including those as a wife, mother, doula, trainer, and leader of others. I was touched, forever changed, and my spirit was lifted.

Who knew that at this non-birth conference I would be most affected by a story of birth? You see, one of the general session speakers shared her very personal, very intimate birth story with me and about 8,000 others in attendance. She shared her first two births, both beautiful and amazing, one a twin birth. She shared a little insight into her world with three sweet little daughters, the challenges of mothering toddlers and small children, and eventually her experience preparing for her growing family of 6. Her name is Angie and her story is one that has the ability to reach deep down and touch us in the depths of our souls. As she spoke, I cried.

I'd like to tell you a little of the story that I heard on this day, as it changed the way I look at joyful birth. It is a journey that is packed full of emotion, love, deep sadness, faith, and eventually joy. The speaker and her family (husband and three daughters) were eagerly anticipating the arrival of newest daughter. They were doing all of the preparations that most new parents do, and they were all gaining excitement as the pregnancy progressed. Around 20 weeks pregnant, they received the no-doubt gut wrenching news that their new baby would likely not survive. They were given little hope as to her ability to live, with major organs being affected, or not developing in a way that would sustain life outside of the womb. As we listened to her story, we were all in tears with her. Many of the 8,000 women in that room were mothers too; some had lost babies of their own, and even those who weren't could relate to some of the fears and anxieties that she expressed. One thing that struck me was her ability, her necessity to hang onto her faith through her painful journey.

As this mother described what was important to her as she coped with the circumstances surrounding her impending birth, I was immediately struck by her expression of joy. I asked myself, *how is it possible that she could find joy in what must have been the most painful experience of her life?* I began to truly think about the possibility for joyful birth to include all kinds of birth, no matter the outcome. As her story continued, I also continued to examine the emotions surrounding birth in general, and my own preconceived notions. For just a moment I tried to think of how I would handle it if I were ever in her shoes. Would I even be able to get out of bed in the morning?

She told us all of trips that her family took with baby before her birth to cherish each and every moment that they had with her. I was breathless to learn that this family decided to *share life* with their unborn child, knowing that they would not be sharing their whole lives with her after she was born. As a birth professional, I ask (myself and others), *do we really appreciate the mother/baby bond even before birth?* I found an entry from this mother on her blog that I felt was really touching:

> "We settled into the reality of 'our new life,' and the stacks of books on pregnancy gave way to scripture. Did you know that while you were in my tummy, you went to the beach, to Disney World, to the ballet, to the zoo, to the symphony, to pick out our puppy, to the children's theater, to listen to daddy sing, to church, to Poppy's house ... and so many more places. I talked to you about how the laundry machine

worked, told you about all our neighbors, and taught you how to choose a ripe pineapple at the grocery store. I never stopped talking to you. You were my daughter, and I loved you like I love your sisters. We prayed for you all the time."

This family knew that they only had this baby for a short time … and they reacted by doing with their baby in utero what many parents strive to do with their children every day; they taught their daughter about the world around them and how to live in it! Wow!

Some research suggests that when a baby is not going to live or perhaps has already passed, if possible allow the mother to hold her baby after birth. We know that sometimes the act of holding the baby helps a mother find closure. What this family did with their time with their new baby encompassed so much more than holding her after birth to say goodbye. They lived *with* her while she was alive. What I learned from that very act was that there is no one right way to cope with infant loss. What some people might have found as too painful to even think about brings others comfort.

As I listened and learned from this mother, she discussed the steps that her family took to make the upcoming birth and death as peaceful as possible. It was much like how many moms prepare for birth, except she didn't take evening primrose oil, walk, or drink raspberry leaf tea. She prepared heart and soul to say hello and goodbye in one breathless moment. Although the family prayed for a miracle, it did become clear at some point that it was not likely. The doctors told this family they would have their baby for about 2 minutes once she entered this world.

And here's where the joy really shone through: When she discussed her time with her precious newborn after her cesarean birth, she focused on the very precious time that she had with her both inside her womb and out, rather than her loss. She shared her *joy* and yes, she used that word, when her daughter lived for 2.5 hours, not 2 minutes. She shared the joy in realizing that her daughter weighed in at 3 pounds 2 oz, not 2 pounds as predicted. She said, *"My daughter had weight in this world."* Is it possible that this 2.5 hours was actually filled with joy for this family? Is it possible that mothers all over the world can find joy in a birth that also brings so much emotional pain?

On the day I heard Angie speak about her joys and her pain, I was brought to sobbing tears. What happened in that arena full of 8,000 women still takes my breath away. As it turns out, it happened to be the national day of remembrance for pregnancy and infant loss. In honor of this day, doing something she had not done before at this conference, the speaker asked those that were willing, and who had experienced a loss of a pregnancy, infant or child, to stand in remembrance. This is where the world stopped. In each direction, I was surrounded by standing women. Although we'll never know how many women stood, I would estimate that at least half, guessing 4,000-5,000 women. They represented at least one child whom they no longer held. In my own group, a dear family member stood, honoring the babies that she had also lost. As she stood, and I sat, we held hands and cried. The message to the standing women and to those of us still sitting was simple: *Your babies held weight in this world.*

As a doula, I am well aware of the very important issue of pregnancy and infant loss. I know that all too many times, our clients and other mothers experience the deep sadness with the loss of a baby, a dream. But as a doula, I had not before considered that for some, joy plays a part of their story as well. You see, I thought that I, for one, and many of my other doula sisters, knew what a "joyful birth" really looks like. But in reality, each woman can find her own joy in her own birth. It was in hearing this story of joyful loss that I truly began to understand that each baby, those here on earth and those who have left us for heaven, bring joy. And while yes, no matter what the babe's age or gestation, there certainly is a sense of loss and absolutely a need for mourning, but let us not forget to leave room for joy.

What does a joyful birth look like? I've learned that it's different for you, for me, and for the women in our care. Much like love itself, it has no bounds, and it has many faces.

This year, I am honored to say that I was privileged to bear witness to joyful birth in many different forms. I watched as women found their voice in their birth, found their place in birth, and found their joy in birth. It is through all of them that I experienced what is truly uniquely, joyful birth.

(To learn more about Angie's story, her family or her book *I Will Carry You*, please visit: www.angiesmithonline.org)

The Point of No Return

by Jana Lok

MY FIRST BIRTH EXPERIENCE WAS not all in the way that I had imagined. Early on, I had decided that I wanted a natural birth. I was determined to go medication-free and, ideally, give birth in my own home. Shortly after becoming pregnant, I sought out the services of the local midwifery practice. Now came an even more important task, to find the perfect doula. I had not had any real experience with a doula. I first learned about doulas when my nephew was born. His mother had sought the guidance of a doula, and although I didn't know the particulars of her labor and delivery, both she and my brother were happy to have her there. Even as I progressed through nursing school, there wasn't much discussion about doulas and the importance of their role. Years later, once I had completed graduate school and was teaching, I found out that one of my colleagues had been a doula before she became a nurse. She inspired her students to become more holistic practitioners.

Unfortunately, by the time that I became pregnant, she was no longer practicing but recommended me to a doula who became one of the most important people in my childbirth and post-partum journey. The first time we met, I knew that she was the perfect doula for me. She exuded confidence and a sense of calmness that immediately drew me in. She was highly experienced, and yet respected the uniqueness and newness of my own pregnancy. My husband was also delighted with her. She was the first person who called us a family so early on in the pregnancy.

As my pregnancy was coming to an end, she asked me to come up with a birth plan. Although I had briefly discussed some preferences with my midwifery team (for example, no medication, no artificial rupturing of membranes), now I had the opportunity to really reflect on the things that were important to me during birth. A week later, I had finished writing my "Home Birth Plan." I included information about my labor, birth companions, pain relief, birthing position, and aftercare of the baby. Ironically, the labor and delivery was almost everything but what I had envisioned! Yet, having the plan in the back of my mind certainly gave me more focus and clarity during labor.

My pregnancy had gone smoothly thus far. I was energized, still finding time to get exercise and take long walks with the dog. I had few aches and pains, hadn't experienced any Braxton Hicks contractions or other pregnancy-related discomfort. My husband and I were gearing up for a home birth. Everything was set. We had brought the home-birthing kit from the midwifery clinic, and I had collected all the recommended birthing accessories (extra sheets, blankets, space heater, and more). I was planning to labor in my tub and either have a water-birth or deliver in my bed.

My due date came and went. I was starting to feel anxious. I saw my midwife on my fortieth week and she started planning my post-dates management. As per policy, the following Monday, she scheduled me for an non stress test at the local hospital. Following that test, I was to have a biophysical profile ultrasound done. On Wednesday that week, she booked me for a gel placement, which would be followed by an induction on the Thursday morning starting at 9 a.m.

During this time, I had daily phone conversations with my doula. She became the sounding-board of my fears and anxieties. She helped me focus my thoughts and prepare myself mentally for my labor. I had so many unfinished graduate-school projects looming over me, and my husband was working extra-long hours and in the midst of changing jobs. I hadn't given myself much time to slow down and really concentrate on this important and life-changing event. I think that my body knew that I wasn't ready. My doula helped me channel these thoughts, and she was integral in getting me to let go of things that I could not change and get mentally ready to welcome my child. She assured me that once I was ready, things would fall into place.

Perhaps I was never quite prepared, as with most new parents. Aside from feeling some very mild contractions while out on brisk walks with my dog, nothing was happening. That Monday as scheduled, my husband and I arrived at the hospital for the non stress test. We were escorted to a small room and I was hooked up to a fetal monitor. About an hour later, things were not looking great. They expected to see a number of fetal heart rate accelerations during the monitoring period and the baby did not respond as predicted, ticking away at a steady 140 bpm the whole time. They immediately sent me for an ultrasound.

I was starting to get really worried. I was even more alarmed when the ultrasound technician made an off-hand remark about whether we had undergone the integrated prenatal screening test, and how large the baby seemed. The technician handed me the report to bring back to the unit. I glanced at it quickly. Sometimes being a healthcare provider has its disadvantages. The report showed a grade 4 placenta, increased nuchal translucency, and a weight estimate for 10 pounds 8 ounces. My anxiety levels were through the roof! I was so worried about the health of my baby and also about the possibility that baby might be born with complications. The hospital paged my midwife with the results of the tests. After consulting with the obstetrician, she told me that it would be best if they induced me as soon as possible.

Everything seemed surreal. I was thinking that this would be a routine test and that we would sit and wait for a few more days until the baby was ready to arrive. Suddenly, my vision of a quiet and uncomplicated home birth was turning into a hospital nightmare I had never envisioned. I called my doula and explained the situation. She asked me when I wanted her to come. I had no idea how things would progress and I really wanted her with me as soon as possible.

My midwife examined me and determined that I was about 1 centimeter dilated. She was certain that I would have gone into labor any day now. She also said it was a good sign and that the induction would likely proceed quite smoothly.

A few hours later, I sat in a hospital bed wearing the traditional blue-spotted hospital gown, an IV was running in my right hand, and a fetal monitor was strapped across my abdomen. This was not the vision I had of my labor. I remember a number of times that my doula had asked to think about how I imaged my labor would be. She would ask me to use all of my senses in thinking about the experience. Well, here I was in a cold, private birthing room. The pale, earth-toned walls were softened by a handful of small light fixtures. There were monitors beside my bed, and an array of hospital furniture. I was feeling frightened, and anxious. I could hear the humming of the motor on the IV pump next to me, and I still felt the faint after-burning of having had an IV jabbed in my hand. I was also feeling the tightness of the fetal heart-rate monitor strapped across my abdomen. I could smell the disinfectant laden hospital air. This was definitely a far cry from my comfortable home and the place where I expected to meet my baby.

My husband had left to pick-up a few things from the house seeing as we hadn't packed anything.

For the next few moments, I was mostly alone. A few times a midwife or her student would come by to see how I was doing. They were able to monitor my contractions remotely from the nurses' station, so in my early labor, there wasn't much interaction between myself and my healthcare team.

I was very happy to see my doula when she arrived. Her inherent calmness eased my anxiety. I remember almost apologizing for me not being able to deliver at home like we had planned. She asked me how I was feeling, and it was reassuring for me to be able to share my concerns. Shortly thereafter my husband returned bringing some things from home. We had also ordered some food from the local Indian take-out. I was feeling better at this point. The contractions had started, but they were not really causing me any pain more like tightening sensations in my abdomen. Another friend of mine also arrived for support. In the next hour, we enjoyed light conversation and delicious butter chicken with naan!

The midwife was checking on me periodically as they adjusted the dose of the picotin. Gradually, the intensity of the contractions began to increase. I started to feel pain in my cervix, a dull ache that progressed into an intense, sharp pain. I now needed to focus all my attention to what my body was doing. My doula was right there through every contraction. She helped me focus my breathing, and kept encouraging me along the way. Even though I was on the monitor and limited in my movement, she suggested trying other positions. I tried lying, standing, and sitting on a birthing ball. At one point, the midwife agreed to let me take a warm shower to ease the discomfort. I found that I felt the most comfortable sitting straight up in the bed with my legs crossed right under me. My doula kept talking to me. I found this most reassuring especially when I was no longer able to verbalize my feelings. She massaged my lower back, and eased the tension out of my shoulders. She encouraged me to relax my upper body and breathe through every contraction. She became my guide; I was entirely focused on her voice, and followed each of her suggestions with the best of my ability. Even though the pain was becoming almost unbearable, I felt in control.

The midwife wanted to check my progress. As soon as I lay down, the intensity of the contractions became unbearable. I lost my focus. Inside, I wanted to scream, but only let out a faint groan. I was about 7 centimeters dilated now. The midwife wanted to rupture my membranes. She had wanted to do this earlier on, but I had declined as I had read that it could greatly increase the intensity of the contractions. I was so determined to have a natural childbirth, again, I declined.

Now, all of my effort was spent getting through each contraction. They had become so frequent that I barely had time to recover. At one point, the midwife entered the room saying that she was turning off the picotin as my contractions were literally one on top of the other. Yes! I was thinking to myself, I know that, I can certainly feel them! Somewhere around this time, my friend left. I still sensed my husband near my side, but my world was comprised of nearly unbearable pain, and the one person who was guiding me every step of the way, my doula.

The intense pain persisted for about two more hours, and then suddenly, I was starting to feel an intense urge to push. The midwife checked me again. She said that she was feeling my membranes bulging and this time I consented to her rupturing them. I felt a warm rush of fluid. She said that I still needed to progress and I was not to push.

This was the most difficult part of the labor. Every part of my body was saying to push, I was unable to fight this feeling. I grunted. Tears were streaming from my face. My body made me push at the end of each contraction and I was unable to hold back. I was shaking. I felt that I had lost all control. Again, my doula was right there. She held my hand. At this point, I wasn't hearing any words, but I felt her presence.

It was around 1:00 a.m. when the midwife finally announced that I was fully dilated and to start pushing with each contraction. I was so exhausted by now. Yet, actively trying to push with each contraction offered some relief. I became aware that the end was approaching. Soon I would be holding my new baby. I was listening to the midwife's directions and pushing as hard as my body would let me.

For 90 minutes I struggled. Then, there was some commotion. Apparently, the baby was starting to get distressed. The next few moments were a blur. The OB was called. A high-flow oxygen mask was placed on my face. People began entering my room: nurses, respiratory technicians, and finally the OB. I was positioned flat on my back, my knees were being held and pushed toward my head. I felt a pricking sensation of the local anaesthetic being injected, and then I had the realization that I was getting an epi-siotomy. I felt out of control. Separated from my own body, and no longer an active part of this process. Yet, my doula stayed right there. Although she could not change the progression of events, it was comforting for me that she was there, witnessing this, and knowing that one day, we could again revisit this and work through it together.

The baby was born on the second push along with the assis-tance of the vacuum device. I felt the child being pulled right out of me. There were moments of tension in the room as the baby was born, and then a sense of relief that everything was fine. We had a healthy new baby. My husband was able to cut the umbili-cal cord. As the baby was placed on my chest, my husband spoke these words which will forever be ingrained in my memory, "You got your wish, it's a girl!" Well, my wish was really for a healthy baby, and in the end that is what matters the most.

My labor and delivery did not go like anything I had expected or even imagined. Sometimes when I think back, I occasionally feel that there were things I could have done differently. I begin to doubt myself. I felt that my body had let me down. It has been my doula who has offered gentle words of encouragement. She has been my sounding-post in my moments of doubt. She has given me the greatest complement that any parent could get: she's called me an amazing mother. She has seen things that my own family has not seen. She has shared my fears, comforted me when I experi-enced the most intense pain that I had ever known, and reassured me every time that I ever doubted myself. She has witnessed and shared the most important day of my life: the day that I became a mother. She has given me the confidence to know that even though things don't go according to plan, I worked to give my daughter the best start to her life.

In the spring of 2010, I got pregnant with my second child. My daughter was only 10 months old. My pregnancy with her and her birth were still very much fresh in my mind. She had provided us with challenges right from her first day when she decided not to latch for breastfeeding. She didn't care to sleep very often or for very long periods of time, and cried incessantly. I think that my friends and family were quite surprised when my husband and I decided to have another baby in quick succession. I figured we already hadn't been sleeping much in the last few months, how much more difficult could another baby really be? Yet, my biggest trepidation was in facing another traumatic labor and delivery.

Following my daughter's birth, I felt that my body had failed me. I had a difficult physical recovery as well, healing from a third degree tear. I had felt physically and emotionally depleted, not at all an ideal way to begin caring for a new life. Yet, somehow we got through those difficult first few months. I recovered physically. I owe a significant part of my emotional healing to my doula. She stayed in close contact with me for many weeks following my daughter's birth. She provided on-going breast-feeding support and connected me with the very best resources available. We had many conversations about my labor and delivery. She helped me express my feelings and truly come to terms with the experience. However difficult it was, in the end I had received the best gift of all, a beautiful and healthy baby girl.

One day mid-May, I remember calling my doula shortly after learning that I was pregnant for the second time. I was quite excited to share this news with her. She remarked how she hadn't had a doubt that I would have another baby. She was really happy for me. I asked her again to be my doula. I also mentioned that I hope that this experience would be a lot different from the last. She assured me that it would. I truly love her optimism!

We kept in close contact during my pregnancy. While I was pregnant with my daughter, I had felt wonderful. This time things were a lot different. I felt more tired. I started getting back and joint pain. I had a lot of round ligament pain, and felt extreme pressure on my cervix. I had difficulty maintaining an active lifestyle.

I told my doula that I wanted to do everything possible to avoid another induction. She assured me that this time I would have my home birth and things would progress naturally. My baby was due mid-January. By December, I was starting to feel extremely uncomfortable. I would get frequent Braxton Hicks, and because I had never experienced these in my last pregnancy, I started to think that perhaps this baby would come early.

With my last pregnancy, my doula had said that the baby would come when I was truly ready, both mentally and physically. I had had a lot on my mind recently. At the beginning of December, I had successfully completed my PhD proposal defense and that had certainly taken a huge weight off my shoulders. With most of my academic work now completed, I just had a few research projects that I needed to hand in and then I could really focus on the birth of the baby.

My doula was going away on holidays around Christmas time, and although she had made arrangements for a back-up doula, I was really anxious about her not being here should I go into labor. I promised her that I would wait for her to come back! I was relieved when the New Year came and she contacted me to let me know that she had returned.

I once again began planning for my home birth. I brought my home birthing kit from the midwifery clinic. I collected all the necessary items that the midwives recommend for a home birth. I had everything organized in my master bedroom. I was hoping to labor in my room or my bath-tub and either have a water-birth or deliver on my bed.

As my due date approached, the midwives decided to do a "stretch-and-sweep" to hopefully get things going. They did one at 39 weeks and another at 40 weeks with no result. We were both trying to avoid going post-dates given what happened last time. I tried to do some walking and keep active even though I was much more uncomfortable than the last time. I was also having nerve pain down one leg that would occasionally cause numbness. I went to see a chiropractor a few weeks before my due date and I had found it helpful in relieving my discomfort.

My due date came and went yet again. I started to feel anxious and began researching other ways of trying to induce labor. I was also a little worried that I wouldn't recognize when I had gone into labor since my first had been induced. One evening at 2 days past my due date, I hauled out the breast pump and put it to work. I'm not sure if that truly did the trick, or whether my body decided to conform to the statistical norm of second babies being born on average three days late, but the next morning something was definitely going on!

I had had bouts of insomnia with this pregnancy, but this morning it was quite different. I remember waking up around 4:00 a.m. and not being able to fall back asleep. I stayed awake for about 2 hours, and then I drifted off for only a short stretch. It was a Saturday morning. A beautiful, but cold January day. My daughter was spending the weekend with my parents, so it was just my husband and me and our big, sappy, yellow lab.

Around 8:00 a.m., my husband and I got up. He decided to go off to the gym for a few hours. I remember nagging at him briefly about not tidying up his papers and stuff in the bedroom. I had been meticulously collecting all the birthing supplies and trying to prepare everything, and was getting irritated by all of his things lying around the room (for example, bills, letters, cables, computer accessories). I decided when he left that I would try to organize the room a little better.

We were also in the midst of a basement renovation. The project was to have been completed early in the new year, but permits had gotten delayed and now everything was set back a few weeks. We weren't enjoying living in a construction zone. I wasn't able to get the nursery set-up. Maybe this was one of those unfinished events that was preventing me from being mentally ready to have this baby!

Shortly after my husband left, I started feeling contractions, although they didn't really feel any different from the Braxton Hicks I had been feeling for many weeks now. I continued trying to organize some things around the house. I started to notice that the contractions were occurring with some regularity. I decided to pull out my laptop and try to find a website I found to keep track of my contraction pattern. My techie husband would certainly applaud this move!

It was around 9:00 a.m. I was now having contractions about every 7 to 9 minutes. I looked at my binder from the midwife clinic and read over the list of symptoms that warranted a page to my midwife; one of them was regular contractions every 5 minutes. I didn't quite meet the criteria so I decided to wait a little longer. I decided that there was a strong possibility that I might go into labor so I began to prepare my room. I lined my bed with a waterproof cover and covered it with old sheets. I got all the birthing supplies lined up on my dresser.

Around 10:00, I knew that things were definitely happening. I sent my husband a text message asking him to come home directly after the gym. My contractions were now getting stronger, and they were still not entirely regular. I wasn't certain of what to do. Should I page the midwife? I was beginning to feel a little anxious. I was home alone. I needed to calm myself, I needed to focus. I called the one person who I felt could offer me what I needed right then. I called my doula.

A few minutes later the phone rang and it was her. It was a great relief hearing her voice on the phone. I told her that things were definitely happening. She shared my excitement. She had been anticipating my call. I smiled. Everything was falling into place. I was beginning this labor on a beautiful and crisp January morning. I felt invigorated, but more importantly, I left in control and was ready to trust my body. I told her that my contractions were now about 6 to 8 minutes apart and lasting for around 45 seconds. I had also noticed some pink discharge earlier. I mentioned that my husband was at the gym and would be home soon. She asked me if I had paged the midwife. I had not.

We agreed that that was the next step. She told me that she would get ready and then call me again when she was on her way. I was a little nervous when she said she would be arrive in about 1 to 2 hours as I had no idea how quickly I might progress. I'm not sure if she sensed my anxiety, or if she just knew that I needed her to be there as soon as possible, but she made the drive from midtown to my suburban home with due haste!

After getting off the phone with my doula, I again hesitated. Was I really in labor? The nature of the contractions hadn't really changed, and there was still no precise pattern. I again continued to track them on the computer. Suddenly a few contractions came about 3 minutes apart. Shortly after 11:00, I paged the midwife. Two minutes later, a midwife whom I had not met previously returned my page. She introduced herself and apologized that my team members were not able to be on-call this morning as they had been at another birth overnight. I described my symptoms. I was still sitting on a birthing ball in my bedroom near the edge of my bed. I found that the counter-pressure exerted by the ball really helped with the escalating pain. She wanted to stay on the phone with me during a contraction so she could evaluate how I was doing. I was coping quite well. I calmly told her when the next contraction started, breathed through it, and told her when it was over. She didn't seem particularly worried, but she said that she would come by to assess me shortly.

My husband arrived home shortly afterwards. I was still coping well, remaining perched on my ball. I asked him to get some things ready and told him that the midwife and doula were en route. My contractions were now between 3 and 5 minutes, lasting between 30 to 45 seconds.

I was elated when my doula arrived. Here I was as we had planned and discussed: laboring in my home, having gone naturally into labor. In a few hours, I would be welcoming a baby in my home. No hospital, no medication and no unnecessary interventions. I would let my body do its work. She asked me how I was doing. She helped me breathe through my contractions. The pain was getting to be more intense.

The midwife arrived shortly after noon. By now, my contractions were getting to closer to 3 minutes apart, lasting for 45 seconds. She asked me to lie on the bed to examine me. The position change caused quite a bit of discomfort. All of a sudden the intensity of my contractions increased drastically. The midwife was also shocked to find that I was already 7-8 centimeters dilated! She panicked a little, and immediately began paging for a second midwife to come.

The doula asked me if I wanted to try any other positions. I had wanted to get into my tub, but I was concerned about getting in too early as I had heard that it could slow down labor. Both the doula and midwife assured me that this was not likely. My doula started preparing the bath. At 12:45, I started to make my way over to the bathroom with her assistance. She was meticulous in ensuring that the temperature was just right, and helped me into a comfortable position. I sat down and leaned against the side of the tub.

I was surprised to find that I had actually felt less pain sitting on the birthing ball than being in the water. But I liked the feeling of sitting in the water. It enveloped my body, and helped to ease some of my tension. The doula sat on the edge of the bath, she touched my shoulders, reminded me to relax my upper body and ease through the contraction. She asked me to envision my body doing its work, my cervix dilating, my baby descending into position.

The second midwife arrived. She was one of my regular care providers. It was nice seeing another familiar face. She stayed with me for a few contractions, complemented me on how I was coping, and then left to prepare with the other midwife. My doula stayed by my side. Although I felt in control, it was reassuring having her there.

As the intensity of the pain increased, the more I began to focus on my task. Periodically, the midwife would check in to see how I was progressing. She asked me to change my position, to open up my legs more, to try to facilitate the dilation of my cervix. She tried checking me in the bath, but had a difficult time as my membranes were still intact. Every movement and every intervention seemed to take away from my focus. They encouraged me to drink, but I wasn't thirsty. They wanted me to change positions, but I felt secure sitting where I was, knowing that any movement might tip my balance and cause me to lose focus. My in-laws and nephew had arrived around this time. I remember hearing a commotion downstairs, and my husband went to tend to them for a few minutes. My doula instantly became concerned that there was too much distraction. I remember reassuring her that it was okay if there were in the house. I really appreciated her concern. She understood how important it was for me to maintain my focus. My husband was immediately sent to ensure that the noise and activity would be kept to a minimum. I'm sure that the doula was prepared to politely evict anyone should the need arise!

Now, the midwives wanted to check me again but on the bed. I was not happy about this, and really dreading having to leave the bath. The midwives also wanted me to void before moving back to the bed. In between contractions, they helped me over to the toilet. I couldn't void, I didn't really feel the urge and I hadn't been drinking much all morning. In my excitement, I hadn't even eaten a proper breakfast. I had started eating some bread crisps around mid-morning, but later on had completely lost my appetite.

My position change and movement had escalated the intensity of my contractions. Suddenly, I was overcome with a wave of nausea. I had remembered this from my previous labor. I vomited mostly water. I had learned an important lesson from my previous labor – spicy Indian food is best avoided!

Slowly, between contractions, I was assisted to my bed. I dreaded lying on my back. The pain was unbearable. I began to lose the focus that I had fought so hard to maintain during the last few hours. I covered my eyes, I couldn't bear to let the midwives see the tears streaming down my face. I groaned. I was 9 centimeters by now, my membranes were bulging. The midwife asked if she could rupture my membranes as it would help with the progression of my labor. I consented. At 1:40 p.m., the midwife ruptured my membranes, and again, I felt the warm rush of fluid oozing around me.

Seeing my extreme discomfort from lying on my back, my doula asked the midwife if I could be allowed to change positions. I was helped to turn over to my side. Within moments, I started feeling the uncontrollable urge to push. For a moment, I was afraid again. Last time, I had had to fight this urge for so long. For a brief second, I also thought what if I couldn't push him out by myself? I was again remembering my last birth and began to have doubts about trusting my body. I told myself, I had no choice. I was going to do this! This was the point of no return, and I needed to have faith in myself.

I was relieved when the midwife said that if I felt the urge that I was to go ahead and push. The midwife also cautioned me to listen carefully to her directions on when to push and stop pushing.

As there was also some anxiety about the size of the baby, I was asked to lie on my back again. My knees were drawn up and pushed toward my shoulders to help with the delivery. My doula was right there to support me. She encouraged my husband to be a part of the experience. She got him to lie next to me on the bed, his head nested toward my right shoulder. It was so comforting feeling his presence. His touch was like a physical bond that held us together as we welcomed our new baby into the world. A good friend of mine who I had called earlier that morning had just arrived. She had wanted to be there for the birth of the baby. The doula was again concerned about the level of distraction, but I assured her that she was welcome to stay.

I was told to push hard and I did. I felt some burning, and then the midwife told me that she could see the head. As the baby's head was delivered, she asked me to stop pushing momentarily. Then, with another strong push, I had delivered my baby. I was so relieved.

At 1:59 p.m., my husband and I welcomed the arrival of our second child. For the next few minutes, we lay on the bed, huddled together. We both had tears in our eyes. I remember wanting to immediately sweep up the baby in my arms, but I was reminded that the baby was still attached to the placenta via the umbilical cord. I was content having the baby lie on my abdomen, feeling the warmth of the baby's body. Everyone had been so excited about the actual delivery that no one had checked the gender yet. One of the midwives picked up the baby to take a look: it was a boy! Moments later, my husband cut the umbilical cord, and I got to hold my baby boy in my arms. It was one of the best moments of my life. He had come into this world in comfort of his own home, surrounding by family, my midwives, and our incredible doula. I remember feeling so relaxed and at ease lying on my own bed. My doula stayed with me for a few hours after the delivery. She made sure that I was doing well. She helped me latch my baby for the first time, and we were both excited when he was successfully breastfeeding.

We continued to keep in touch frequently over the next few weeks. On many occasions, we talked about my second birth experience and compared it to my first. It was the most peaceful and beautiful birth that I could have imagined. I couldn't have been more happy. My doula had helped me to make this birth experience truly wonderful. She taught me to believe in myself, trust my own body, and ultimately to allow me to have the birth experience that every woman deserves.

A Gorgeous Natural Birth

by Heather Aguilera

I MET WITH EMILY AND MARK EARLY in their pregnancy and as we spent our first meeting discussing their previous birth experience and their reasons for thinking that a doula might help them have a better experience this time, it became clear that the current mainstream way of birthing may not match the lifestyle that they were leading. I asked them if they had ever considered the services of a midwife, and after explaining how they work, Emily and Mark looked at each other as if to ask why they had never thought of that option. Within a week, they had setup a meeting with midwives and were on their journey toward a birth to be remembered.

Our meetings were happy, exciting, and easy going. On our second prenatal meeting Emily told me that they had begun exploring the option of a homebirth. She was excited about the great new things they were learning. Emily seemed to be gobbling up all the information she could about the social constraints of birth and was amazed by what she was learning. She and Mark watched "The Business of Being Born" and were getting fired up. Mark particularly was shocked by the documentary and was eager to get even more informed. I gave them the name of another documentary, "Pregnant in America," but advised that they watch that one after the baby was born.

We talked a lot of how their daughter Meg was interested in participating in the birth and I assured her that this was wonderful and that there were plenty of ways that she would feel involved. Meg came in and out of our meetings and was excited and confident about the upcoming birth. Diagrams were very helpful to her understanding.

As Emily's due date came and went, she did not come across as too impatient. She let me know that while she was getting very frequent and often strong practice contractions, she was remaining patient. Mark did call me once and left a message to let me know that Emily appeared to be in early labor but as it turned out, it did not progress.

Finally, over a week past due, Mark called me at 2:00 in the morning and let me know that Emily had been having steady contractions for about 7 hours, and although the contractions were still 7 to 8 minutes apart, they were now needing my help. I arrived at their home at about 2:30 a.m. to find Emily lying on the settee in front of the fireplace keeping her back warm and Mark tracking progress on the iPad. She was experiencing discomfort in her back and the heat seemed to help her. After I arrived, the contractions slowed down and Emily was able to sleep a bit between contractions. The contractions at this time were as far as 24 minutes apart and as close as 7 minutes but very manageable. At about 5:00 a.m., Emily felt that everything was under control and that it might be beneficial for Mark to go to bed. He readily complied. Emily and I got up and walked around the house for a while and then at about 6:30 went outside to enjoy the beautiful June morning and a change of scenery. Emily introduced me to her roosters, pig, horses, and rabbits. The dogs followed us up and down the driveway as the roosters scurried around the backyard. Their daughter Meg woke at 7:30, and after being informed by Pappa that Mommy was downstairs with Heather, she immediately came to find us. Emily was still having discomfort in her back and her contractions were 5 to 6 minutes apart consistently. We decided to go in and have coffee and tea and that we would call the midwife at 9:00 since the contractions were now fairly consistently 5 minutes apart and had been for about an hour.

Emily got some relief from sitting on the ball and gently bouncing, but this seemed to slow down her contractions. Since the contractions were now about 7 minutes apart, we decided that we would wait to call the midwife. At 9:45 we went up to the bedroom and Mark, Meg, and I made the bed to get ready. While upstairs the midwife called and spoke to Mark and then to me and was just calling to see if she might come to sweep Emily's membranes but was happy to hear that she had already started into early labor. We agreed that there was no urgency for her to come since it was still very early even though Emily was curious to see if there was any progress.

We all went downstairs back to the kitchen to find something for Emily to eat. The only thing that was appetizing to her was yogurt covered pretzels. At about 11:15 I suggested that Mark and Emily go outside and walk around a bit while I kept Meg company playing the Monopoly game she had started the evening before. The contractions were getting more intense but were still only about 5 minutes apart. Applying pressure on her lower back was helping at this point.

At 12:10 Emily's parents arrived with homemade bean dip and chips as a snack and to see how things were going. They did not stay long. Emily's very close friend called from Buffalo and informed us that she was on her way.

At 1:00 p.m. Emily was feeling tired, frustrated, and anxious to know if she was making any progress at all. She decided that knowing where she was might help so asked Mark to page the midwife. When she called she spoke with Emily for quite some time and then said that the risk of her coming is that Emily would likely be disappointed since she felt that Emily was still early. She came to this conclusion because while she was on the phone with her for 8 minutes, Emily didn't have a contraction and did not sound uncomfortable enough. I spoke with the midwife for a while and informed her that we would continue to try new positions to try to encourage rotation of a baby that may be in the wrong position and causing undue back pain. She asked us to call when Emily's contractions were 3 minutes apart. She also asked if Emily was using the homeopathic products they were given. In fact, Emily thought that she was to use those to start labor and didn't realize that she was to take them once she was already in labor. We immediately started using them.

This telephone call was a bit of a turning point in the emotions of the labor. Emily was clearly upset that the midwife was not coming for a while and we as a team had to work hard to get over this hurdle. She was crying and this was causing some distress to Meg. Emily did not think it was a good idea for Meg to go to her friend's house at this time.

At 1:15 p.m., we reviewed some of the illustrations that I had and Emily and Mark decided to go upstairs to try the hands and knees position on the bed. Emily got good relief in this position and felt that she even dozed a bit between contractions. At one point Meg became visibly upset and ran into her own room. I went to sit with her on her balcony to comfort her and explain some of what was happening while mom and dad stayed in the bedroom.

At 2:30 we all went outside and Meg went swimming. Emily and Mark labored under the patio canopy while I kept Meg company and watched her in the pool. At 4:00 Emily's friend arrived and was a welcome distraction. Emily was hanging onto Mark for many of her contractions, and while the contractions were getting even more intense, they were still 5 minutes apart. Emily was making some noises and this was upsetting Meg: "Can't you stop making that noise and just say Ouch?" This comment had an immediate effect on Emily's behavior and the noises she was making. I suggested to Meg that maybe she could go and spend some time with Emily's friend's daughter. Meg leapt at the opportunity and left.

As soon as Meg left at 5:00, Emily decided to get into the tub. Once upstairs she said something like "Now I can let go." She got into the tub and after just a few minutes her water broke. The contractions immediately intensified and we got her out of the tub and onto the toilet. Mark called the midwife at 5:30 and she said that she was coming right now and that she was also calling the second midwife. Emily labored on her side on her bed holding Mark's hand and keeping a focused gaze on my eyes. I modeled breathing for her and she quickly found her rhythm.

The midwives arrived within minutes of each other at 6:00 pm and determined that Emily was fully dilated and pushing began at 6:30. Emily's parents arrived around this time just to bring us some soup and found us laboring hard upstairs. We tried various positions to try to encourage the baby to descend and get into a better position since the midwives were pretty certain that he was posterior. We tried pushing on hands and knees, side lying, squatting facing the head board, sitting on the birthing stool, and finally got the best results with Emily on her back.

Emily was working so hard with Mark and me at her side. The midwives kept saying that she was so close and that they could see the baby but after hearing that for over half an hour, the words no longer had much effect. While I whispered and counted down pushes to Emily in her ear, Mark started nipple stimulation at the midwife's suggestion to increase the strength of the contractions.

Meg called to find out how things were going and was told that the baby was coming soon so she wanted to come home. She arrived at about 8:30. She was a very welcome addition to the scene in the bedroom. The midwives told her that they could see the baby. Her response was: "If you see him again, grab him!" Her encouragement and outward displays of love and pride in her mom were remarkable. I think that her presence was a great motivation for her mom since, after 2 hours of pushing, the baby arrived just 20 minutes after his sister came into the room.

Emily's friend was a great support offering verbal prompting and taking lots of photos without being intrusive. Emily's mother was also wonderful with her quiet presence and willingness to help as needed and wiping Emily's forehead, chest and back of her neck with cold, damp cloths.

The baby was born posterior with the cord wrapped twice. This had no negative effects on the baby, and he pinked-up quickly and cried immediately. He was beautiful in every way and was very interested in the breast right from the start. During my last prenatal visit, Emily had expressed to me that once the initial postpartum moments had passed, she would be content for someone else to take the baby and hold him. When the time actually came though, she held on tight and could not stop crying and laughing. They stayed together for a long time before Mark took over.

This was a spectacular birth and had so many noteworthy elements that played on its success. First and most importantly was Emily and Mark's faith in the process and this came predominantly from educating themselves. This was extremely valuable and allowed them to get through the pregnancy, going past due and a long early labor. They hired me and that was an additional source of information and seemed to help get through a couple of hurdles in the labor itself. The most exciting factor that played on their labor was Meg herself. In discussion before the birth, the family agreed that Meg would be at the birth but only if she felt comfortable. Emily expressed concern about Meg's sensitivity. What we saw clearly as the labor progressed was that at some point Meg was outside her comfort zone and needed to leave so that the labor could progress and then later Meg had to come back so that she could give her mom the extra strength she needed to push the baby out.

This is a family that is very in tune with each other and now they have another member to be woven into the fabric of their lives. It was an absolute joy to participate in preparing for and welcoming the arrival of this beautiful boy. I am so thankful that I was invited to be a part of it.

Birth Starts and Ends With Love

by Nicole McKay

IT WAS MID-AFTERNOON ON A weekend when the phone rang. It was my client Shelly, a very petite woman with a beautiful smile that could light up the room. She cheerfully told me that her contractions were getting closer together. She and her husband would like me to meet them at home in about an hour.

I arrived and was greeted with a warm hug and was able to see Shelly experience a few contractions. Josh had been timing them and the pattern seemed to have changed. Shelly walked back and forth between the kitchen and the living room, finding the most relief when she was walking during the contractions. Sometimes she would lean against the counter or table and sway for a moment and then resume her walking. Between contractions, we spoke about the recent weeks, our families, and shared some laughs.

Josh made some food and we all sat together and ate. Shelly occasionally got up and walked to ease her contractions. Noticing the contractions were still a little unpredictable and spaced out, we talked about some acupressure points that could help. Josh held the ones in her hands and me the ones inside her ankles. After only a few contractions, we seemed back on track. Keeping our momentum, I suggested we take a walk outside. It was a grey day with a very light mist – Shelly's favorite weather. Josh helped her put on her rain boots and we took a long walk together, feeling the wind and the quiet of a Saturday afternoon. Shelly's contractions continued as we walked and she was still smiling albeit focused on the great energies of her body.

We made a few quick stops on our walk – the first at a store to print some pictures of her cousin's baby she wanted to take with her and the second, to pick up some dry cleaning. No one knew the magic that walked among them that day in the mall. Her body was working on bringing forth a new life in the world.

A few more hours at home, as the sun was leaving the sky for the day, Shelly and Josh decided that it was time to go to the hospital where they planned on birthing their baby. As is the usual procedure, she had an exam in triage. The doctor said she was 3.5 centimeters dilated and Shelly was crushed. It had been hours! We left triage for some walking of the hospital halls. In one of the hallways, Shelly looked at me with tears in her eyes. She didn't want the news she just had upstairs. I talked to her and Josh reassuringly – her body knows what it is doing and we are going to help it along. Her body can birth her baby because it is already working on it, doing what it needs to do.

We walked down to the cafeteria to get some water and then back down the halls to a large waiting room. Shelly decided she'd like to be in the clothing she packed, which was made for her with lots of love. The gown she packed was handmade by her grandmother, who had passed away about a year before. Bright and colorful. Because she had already experienced a few strong contractions, I helped her change into her gown in the bathroom. The gown brought her grandmother into her space.

I could see on her face that her contractions had somehow changed. She no longer greeted them with a smile. I asked her during the next contraction to see her body hugging her baby – that's all the contractions were for her, just little baby hugs. We spoke to Liam, the name they had chosen for their son, who was wiggling his way into the world. I encouraged to her talk to him – we must have been in that bathroom for at least 30 minutes. Shelly spoke nothing but words of love for Liam.

We returned to Josh in the empty waiting room. Shelly enjoyed slow dancing at this point in her labor. Sometimes she would lean on Josh, sometimes she would lean on me. Together the three of us danced to the music of her body. Few words were exchanged here; we all knew that there was so much power in those moments. We did convey what we needed to with touch, which speaks straight from the heart. We wanted Shelly to know that she was doing something amazing, powerful.

Shelly broke the quiet of the night when she said she thought her water broke. A stream of clear amniotic fluid ran down her leg and onto the floor. Her labor was certainly progressing well. The intensity increased for Shelly, but it was never more than she could handle. We held her in our arms, massaged her back, and reminded her that Liam was on his way and would soon be in her arms.

We slowly made our way back upstairs to triage, where we waited some time for an exam. Shelly was starting to feel sick. I grabbed an empty bucket and we lovingly held her hair back. All we had to do was be there in the moment with her and surround her with unconditional love. We danced some more until the doctor came back. Shelly was imagining a flower gently opening; in reality, this flower was her cervix. Shelly told me that this flower was yellow, which made me able to visualize one too. This time, he had great news for Shelly – in only a few hours she had progressed to 9.5 centimeters!

As we walked down the hall into the birthing suite, she began to feel the urge to push. The nursing staff welcomed Shelly, Josh and I as we helped her up onto the bed. Shelly wanted to use the squat bar, and with gravity on her side, she brought that baby down quickly. Before we knew it, the doctor was called in to catch the baby. Liam slipped easily into the world and was quickly placed upon Shelly's chest.

Tears filled that birthing room as Shelly held him close, as Josh celebrated his wife and new son, and as I watched the three of them get to know each other.

I left the hospital that night, looking up at the moon in the sky, breathing in the fall air, and knowing that love created Liam and it was love that brought Liam into the world.

Shifting Perspective

by Barbara Pal

WHETHER BIRTH IS JOYFUL OR NOT depends on a kaleidoscope of factors: the mental, emotional, and physical preparation of the birthing mother, the perspective of the birthing mother and her partner, the attitudes of her healthcare providers, and the particular circumstances of her birth.

I am constantly amazed at the different things women bring to birth with themselves, and how they respond to the challenge of labor. As a doula, I am always learning something new about a style of care, about human interaction, about support, and about people. Women bring a unique history, physiology, belief system, values, experiences and a genetically unique baby to birth. This is why I don't believe in comparing one woman to another – "Well, SHE could do it, why not HER?" Each woman faces labor and birth with her own unique perspective and challenges. I prefer walking with a woman from where she is at and supporting her education and choices based on where she is at.

Laboring women never cease to surprise or amaze me. At one birth early in my doula career, a young immigrant woman with a Buddhist background labored quietly, peacefully, breathing evenly.

When we got to the hospital and learned she was in transition, I couldn't believe it. Surrendering to the support the midwives, her partner and I provided her, she never felt afraid because she calmly accepted that "this work just has to be done," and knew that we would all be there for her when she needed us. She and her partner planned a homebirth, but ended up transferring to hospital due to meconium in the fluid. She labored there for a long time and pushed for hours. Finally, a caesarean was recommended and she calmly accepted it. I was very surprised because we had met several times and prepared so thoroughly for a natural birth. It was eye-opening to me how much attitude affects a woman's experience of birth. I was permitted to attend the caesarean and enjoyed the playful attitude of the nurses and doctors on staff that evening. They offered radio music to my client during the surgery, any station she wanted. She chose rock and roll. I helped her get information from the anesthesiologist when she felt uncomfortable sensations due to the epidural. When her baby was being born, the obstetrician said, "Okay, get the camera ready!" and I snapped the baby's picture at the moment of his birth. The new mother was so happy to see her baby's face when they placed him next to her. Her partner became teary as he held his son skin-to-skin for the first time. It was a lesson on how being at birth changes men too, from the partners they are to the fathers they become. They fall in love with their baby at birth too. It's quite beautiful, vulnerable and a very personal experience we are witnessing as doulas.

Another time I worked with a moody teenager who was living at home with her parents and younger siblings. Her parents built a tiny private bedroom for her in their small home. I was struck by how grounded and supportive her parents were. They accepted the situation, provided love and guidance for their daughter. At the same time, her parents clearly defined the expectations around whose responsibility it was to care for her baby. During our prenatal visit, the determined teen told me she wanted to have a natural birth without drugs. Her mother had birthed three babies naturally. She worked hard during labor and accepted the hard work. Her labor slowly built to a crescendo. At transition, this young woman was seriously roaring and thrashing loudly. It really helped her take it one contraction at a time, and she used nitrous oxide, which seemed to help her relax. She later told me she was hoping no one would offer her an epidural, because even though it was incredibly intense, she wanted to do it naturally. For this young woman, the joy of birth was finding the power within herself to meet the physical, mental, and emotional challenges of labor, and to accomplish this rite of passage. Right after, she said, "I never want to do that again!" But I really think it did something for her sense of self-confidence that she summoned the inner strength to birth the way she wanted to.

Not too long ago I was one of three doulas at a birth. I love doing births with other doulas, we always bring different ideas and strengths to the experience, and teach each other. It's fun. The expectant mother had a natural-childbirth supportive OB and I was curious to see whether the OB was just paying lip-service, only to jump in with interventions galore, or whether this woman would really have a minimally intervention-laden birth. Completely in touch with her body, the confident, healthy woman labored beautifully. She was not afraid to roll her pelvis, vocalize, and move as she needed to during contractions. She listened to the voices of her doulas, shut out the outer world, and went within. Her OB was completely respectful of her wishes to only have a vaginal exam when she felt like pushing. He seemed in awe of her power to birth naturally. He asked questions about the doula techniques we were using and left the room so we could "labor her." It's so nice to work with healthcare providers in the hospital who understand that doulas can contribute important ingredients to a birth – physical comfort, emotional support, helping a woman to surrender, adopt positions to help her baby move down optimally. My favorite was asking if, during pushing, she could push on her side. "Sure," said the OB, "Why?" We discussed how lying on your back to push is the worst position and how other positions open the pelvis, relieve pain, and so on. I felt a little puzzled like, "Seriously? Am I teaching this to the doctor?"

When we pressed acupressure points on her inner ankles during pushing, he asked, "Does that help with the pushing?" Again, I was amazed that this doctor was asking us questions and showing respect for the mother and her doulas, and in awe of this powerful woman's ability to give birth.

When a woman is in active labor or transition, things move along intensely. Commonly, birthing women struggle with a dip in their confidence in their ability to do it. Here doulas play a big role in helping a woman and her partner to recognize the normal pattern of labor, to accept that it's hard work, and to know she *can* do it. It angers me to no end when a nurse or doctor comes by and says, "Ooooh you poor thing, you look soooo unhappy!" My jaw dropped to the floor once when a healthcare provider said this because the woman was having a great labor. She was enjoying herself as she surrendered to the power of labor. Women do not need others to tell them that they are "not doing it right" if they are vocalizing, moaning, rocking, sweating, crying, vomiting, and pacing. Being quiet and polite does not make for "good labor". Labor is messy and vulnerable. You have to be able to go there, to trust the people you're with to let yourself go, and become your animal self. You have to feel like you can go there, and still be surrounded by love and support. Undermining a woman's confidence does not help her go there.

I can understand and appreciate the liability concerns of nurses and doctors when laboring women come into their care, but the regular hospital protocols and procedures make a healthy, normal labor into a "problem." At a birth I attended this summer, the woman wanted to avoid an epidural. We snuck out of the hospital (tsk tsk tsk!) and enjoyed walking, talking, and laughing downtown during early active labor. When we returned to the hospital, the nurse was very cross that the laboring woman had left the hospital to go on a walk. As punishment, she would be checking baby's heart rate *every 15 minutes*! So stay put! If anything happened to the laboring woman, the nurse would have been in so much trouble! Okay, that I can understand. But did something go wrong? No. The laboring woman was fine, her baby was fine, and she enjoyed walking and talking like a normal, healthy laboring woman.

We worked to make the hospital room dark and womb-like, but

every 15 minutes the nurse interrupted by turning the bright lights on, fiddling with the machines, so the focus was on the equipment, paper and numbers, rather than on the birthing woman. These interruptions kept knocking the woman out of her labor land. I was inwardly rolling my eyes thinking, "How can this woman avoid the epidural with all this interruption and monitoring?" (To be fair, this nurse was otherwise very supportive of the mother's coping and laboring.) This mother eventually got an epidural even though she had wanted to avoid one. I brought a mirror for her to watch her baby move his way toward the light from the warm cushy world of her body as she pushed. She was riveted by the sight. The nurses at this point were so encouraging and fun.

I always love asking nurses about their experiences; at this birth one had been a midwife in Africa and had helped deliver 2000 babies! I think that did a lot for her overall complete comfort and confidence in the birthing mother's ability to birth. It was so much fun to watch the mother's eyes and mouth pop open wide when she pushed her baby out into the world. Whoosh! he went, and she said, "What's that?" She later told me that she found the birth to be an empowering experience, that her body was able to do that, and to create a life.

I wish all women could have a subjectively empowering birth experience.

Finding Myself In Birth

by Jessica Cherniak

To my son Dmitri, whose birth changed the course of my life

I LOVED BEING PREGNANT. FOR THE first time in my life I felt I had a real purpose. My body became my friend. I was mindful of everything that went into my mouth. My mind and body became one. I felt connected. I delighted silently with every movement. It was the longest, but happiest 9 months of my life. On my son's 19th birthday I remember thinking that the 9 months waiting for him seemed longer than his 19 years.

I had no concept of what birth was going to look like but I wasn't afraid of it. All I really knew for sure was that I would miss being pregnant. My partner had wanted to try a home birth. That didn't feel right for me. In my 25 year-old mind, I needed to feel safe. Feeling safe meant my laid-back Irish obstetrician, his wife/nurse (once a midwife in Dublin), and my partner to calmly lead me through my 9 months and whatever birth held for me.

After an uneventful 9 months, 3 days shy of my due date, my OB examined me. "You're dilated 3 centimeters and all thinned out," he proudly exclaimed in his endearing Irish lilt. Not really under-standing what this meant, I feasted on a much craved burger that evening and went to bed crampy. I was up every few hours as usual as my bladder now had my baby's head to contend with. Lying back down at 2:00 a.m. I still to this day don't know whether I felt or heard a "pop," which was followed by a very warm tor-rent. It felt wonderful and frightening all at the same time. I took a moment to collect myself and fathom what was happening before I woke my partner. I felt calm. My partner launched in with ques-tions about contractions. I slowly got out of my soaked bed and was quickly greeted with strong contractions every 3 minutes.

We did the middle of the night trek to the hospital with the rec-ommended list of birthing items in tow. I cursed the city for the state of the roads as we bumped and wove the shortest way to the hospital. Sitting was definitely not a position that felt right for me.

I didn't have a "birth plan" because I had no expectations, only a quiet determination to get through each contraction. I had a partner who was uncomfortable with hospitals and medication. He coached me as I breathed through each contraction. Admitted, all I wanted to do was walk. The thought of being numb and confined to a bed was far more frightening to me than labor itself. My claustrophobia decided for me. I would tell myself during the contraction that it was only going to last a minute, and when it was over I would breathe out the word "peace." I looked forward to the moments of "peace" as opposed to anticipating each contraction. Every so often we would break into song, "Don't worry … be happy" as we looped around the hospital corridors.

We definitely wore a groove in the floor. I had a bruise right in the middle of my forehead from leaning against the wall with each contraction. I needed the front of my thighs massaged very firmly as my labor progressed. My partner settled into my rhythm and I felt supported and safe with him.

My first examination after many hours around the halls yielded only "4 centimeters and paper thin." The full 10 centimeters seemed an eternity away. I had a few moments of panic where I doubted my ability to manage this anymore. The unknown, mixed with no sleep, was a scary place for me. My partner, the OB, and I discussed options. The only one that felt right with me was a shot in the bum of Demerol to take the edge off and to continue my marathon walk.

Not long after I was hit with an overwhelming wave of nausea. I found a hand-washing sink in the hallway just in time.. I instinctively knew things had progressed in the hour since my last exam.

For what seemed like an eternity, but was only 20 minutes, I felt like I took leave of the hospital hallway and found a safe place deep inside myself and decided to let go. It was a primordial place, where I was making sounds, but I swear that I wasn't uttering a sound. I trusted that everything was how it was meant to be, and I was riding a big wave in an endless ocean. A transition trance.

A guttural cry snapped me back into to the institutional starkness. I was shocked to find that it was my own cry. An overwhelming sensation to bear down possessed my body. I did not like this feeling. I was finally convinced to lie on my side so I could be examined. Instinctively I knew I was fully dilated. I finally stood again against everyone's wishes. I squatted by the bed as everyone hovered around me. My OB held my hand and allowed me to squeeze it as I pushed reluctantly with each contraction. I didn't like the sensation of bearing down at all. As the head moved down, I was coaxed by my OB to lie on my side for the last few pushes. It was then I noticed two residents waiting to deliver my baby and my OB still holding my hand. My partner was encouraging me to push. He knew how far I had progressed.

The burning sensation of the head crowning was twice as unpleasant as the pushing. The combination of the two made me think for a moment that I do not want to do this anymore. But once my baby's head emerged, my switch of focus was immediate. I reached down to touch his head and was quickly greeted with the rest of his body. I breathed a big "Peace" and welcomed him onto my chest. Despite a room full of people, I had no real concept of others until the baby was in my arms. I focused on his bright, watchful eyes as they delivered the placenta, repaired a small tear, and bustled around the room. My teary partner now became apparent to me and we shared a beautiful moment nestled around the head of our son. I sipped on a cool beer and relaxed. Finally, I was fully present in the room. Finally, I was fully present in life.

Three more natural births followed this one, each one more empowering than the previous one. My partner's continued support taught me how important it is to be completely present and intuitive with a woman in labor.

Becoming a doula became a natural progression from birthing and mothering my own children. My work needed to have the same emotional ups and downs as mothering. It needed to have a real purpose. The transformation that birth can have on women is life changing and must be honored and protected. This is my calling.

Biographies of Our Contributing Authors

Heather Aguilera

Heather has been assisting women in birth since 2005. She has attended approximately 80 births in and around the greater Toronto area. She started her birthing education as a pre- and postnatal fitness instructor but felt drawn to childbirth education. After her certification, she felt that she needed to get more hands-on birth experience so began volunteering weekly as a labor support person at a local hospital. After moving to the Uxbridge, Ontario area, she was certified as a doula and began working with her own clients. She further expanded her skills working as a second attendant for the local midwives.

Elisa Bisgould-Menendian

Elisa and her husband Rafi have two beautiful and joyful children, Jaime and Jonah. Elisa is an elementary school teacher with the Toronto District School Board during the school year and practices as a doula during the summer months. Elisa became a doula with the belief that every woman should be proud of her birth adventure, no matter what path that adventure takes her on. It is her belief that the mother's partner is vital and that that role should be cherished and respected. "Being a doula is good for the soul, you are needed, you are powerful, you are there to witness a miracle, just remember to breathe!" Elisa can be contacted at: peace.baby@ymail.com

Heather Bradley

Heather is a CBI certified labor doula who came to believe in the power of the body through her own birth experiences. She is a La Leche League Leader, Real Diaper Association Circle Leader and board member, home educator, and military spouse, as well as a doula. Heather has had the pleasure of living in Germany and numerous American states. Her affiliation with the military has given her the opportunity to broaden her world views and help families in locations where support is limited. She currently resides in RAF Lakenheath in England with her husband and their three children.

Julei Busch

Julei Busch lives in one of the most multicultural urban centers in the world. Toronto is truly "The Meeting Place" where wisdoms of 150+ cultural groups rub shoulders and co-exist. Wearing a variety of hats as community health activist, mentor, educator, academic researcher, counselor, vibrational medicine practitioner, doula, and parent, Julei has enjoyed sharing the life journeys of her two children and a true abundance of incredible marvelous people. She feels there is no end of wonder and awe in the world and cherishes this precious human life!

Nuala Byles

Nuala entered the entrepreneurial world in 1990 with the launch of Metaphor Inc., specializing in music, entertainment, and lifestyle marketing. In that same year, she was nominated for a JUNO Award for best album cover design. After 10 successful years, BBDO Canada acquired Metaphor, and Nuala reentered the entrepreneurial world as Creative Director with Garage Inc. In 2011 Nuala joined Ogilvy Action as Creative Director and continues to produce breakthrough campaigns for some of the top global brands.

Lisa Caron

Lisa is co-editor of *Bearing Witness: Childbirth Stories Told by Doulas* along with the newest edition to the Bearing Witness book series, *Joyful Birth*. Lisa found her calling while volunteering with pregnant teens in 1996 and has since attended more than 300 births in homes and hospitals as a certified doula in Toronto. To compliment her passion and commitment to foster healthy confident families, Lisa also brings a calm, intuitive ear, and extensive breastfeeding counseling experience to mothers and babies as a certified postpartum doula specializing in depression and anxiety. To strengthen the Toronto birth work community, Lisa hosts conferences facilitated by prominent international speakers. Outside of birth work, Lisa enjoys urban exploration, wide open spaces, and spending time with her family. www.lisacaron.ca

Jessica Cherniak

Jessica Cherniak, PCD (DONA), is the founder of Fourth Trimester in Toronto. She is an experienced birth and postpartum doula and a mother of four. For more than 15 years she has been providing calm and empowering support to expecting and new Toronto families. Jessica eases the transition into the fourth trimester by providing the support and reassurance needed through birth. She provides the guidance needed in order to respond to the needs of the new baby. She assists in establishing breastfeeding, provides emotional and physical help, and teaches the essentials of newborn care. She is passionate about guiding new mothers through this wonderful and overwhelming transition. www.4thtrimester.ca

Raissa Chernushenko

Raissa is a certified shiatsu therapist and infant massage instructor working and living in Oshawa, Ontario, with her husband and two children. A published poet, she is a member of the Writers' Community of Durham Region and is also actively involved in local community theater. A strong dance and acting background led to her fascination with body awareness and healthy movement, as well as the importance of loving and compassionate touch within all of our significant relationships. She teaches shiatsu based self care, couples and family wellness workshops. Contact her through www.handtohearthealing.com.

Jody Cummins-Lambert

Jody is a Birth Doula, HypnoBirthing Practitioner, urban farmer and beekeeper residing in Guelph, Ontario. She was guided to the doula world almost immediately after the joyful birth of her daughter in 2003. The arrival of a new babe into the world never ceases to amaze Jody. www.timelessbirth.ca

Deborah da Silva

Deborah is a Certified Nutritional Practitioner and founder of Nutrition Therapy in Ajax, Ontario. She is married with two handsome grown sons and two beautiful grandchildren. In her nutrition practice, she coaches people to achieve optimal health by promoting healthy lifestyle choices, such as cleansing programs, weight loss, healthy cooking classes, resistance training, and Nordic pole walking classes. She feels that most disease can be changed from the inside out through proper nutrition. She is available to talk about nutrition or instruct a cooking class in group or corporate workshops. Deborah's email is info@nutritiontherapy.ca and phone 905-239-3485. Her website is www.nutritiontherapy.ca.

Joanne Dahill

Joanne Dahill CD(DONA), LMBT (nc#548), is passionate in service to women and their partners as they welcome a new child into their lives. She is honored to be with them at such a precious and sacred time of life. Although she continues to gather new tools and knowledge to place in her "birth bag," she believes that the greatest gift she can offer is to act as a mirror, reflecting to each woman her own strength, wisdom and capacity to trust birth and her own power. She is affiliated with Hypnobabies, Hypnosis for Childbirth, Calm Birth, HUG Your Baby, Baby's First Massage, and www.JourneyofMotherhood.com

Nelia DeAmaral

Nelia has been in the field for over 14 years as a Birth with Yoga teacher, birth doula, author, and workshop facilitator. Her passion is helping women struggling with pre- and postnatal depression and anxiety. In 2010, she started Ontario's first Postpartum Family Support Line, which has helped hundreds of families through peer-based telephone support services. She is also a mother to two spirited and beautiful girls. She can be reached at www.birthwithcare.com or nelia@birthwithcare.com.

Lisa Doran

Lisa Doran, ND, is the co-editor of *Bearing Witness* (2010) and *Joyful Birth* (2012), and the mother of three beautiful and growing young men who were all birthed at home, her third child unassisted into her own hands. She is a midwifery, homebirth, and breastfeeding advocate. She took her doula training with ALACE in 1991 and has been working as a doula since. She is also a naturopathic doctor, in practice since 1997, with a specialty in fertility, pregnancy, and birth. She offers unique services to her patients with the combination of her naturopathic skills and her doula experience. She is specially trained in acupuncture for fertility and acupuncture in pregnancy. Her clinic, Barefoot Health Naturopathic Clinic, is a busy integrated care clinic in Ajax, Ontario. She co-developed and teaches the third-year Introduction to Maternal Newborn Care course at the Canadian College of Naturopathic Medicine and founded the Association of Perinatal Naturopathic Doctors. Lisa has been published in *Midwifery Today* and *Naturopathic Doctors News and Reviews*. She delivers lectures and seminars all over Canada on topics related to birth and naturopathic medicine. Lisa is also an urban farmer, an avid outdoors woman, a fiber artist, and a blooming celtic fiddler. www.barefoothealth.ca

Vicki File

Vicki is a CBI certified labur doula and mother to one awesome little boy. Her own traumatic birth experience spiraled out of control and left her disappointed and wanting to know more. As she researched and studied and questioned, a new passion began to grow. She wanted to get involved, advocate for normal birth, and help women find their empowerment. She decided to change her whole life, and left the world of corporate advertising behind to embark on a new journey as a birth professional in Brantford, Ontario. More inspired with every birth she attends, she has no regrets. www.vickifiledoula.com

Shawn Gallagher

Shawn Gallagher, BA, BCH, is a board certified hypnotist in private practice in Toronto. As a childbirth educator since 1986, she created and teaches the ChildbirthJoy Prenatal Hypnosis Series, training hundreds of expecting parents in self-hypnosis for birth preparation. She also provides advanced training to hypnotists, doulas, midwives, and other healthcare practitioners in the use of hypnosis during birth. As a HypnoFertility practitioner, she uses a combination of hypnosis, Neuro-Linguistic Programming (NLP), and Emotional Freedom Technique (EFT) to help improve outcomes for fertility and other issues. In addition to her experience as a doula and as a midwife, she is the mother to a son and daughter, both born at home. www.childbirthjoy.com

Robin Gray-Reed

Robin is a registered nurse, international board certified lactation consultant, certified doula, childbirth educator, and nurse-midwifery student. Her passion is providing support and information to parents during pregnancy and postpartum, encouraging mindful attachment between parents and children. She believes that love – in all its many flavors – makes a family, and advocates for full equality for all families. She lives in Seattle, Washington. www.mindfulmidwife.com.

Kerry Grier

Kerry was born and grew up in Zimbabwe. She has always loved babies and has accompanied many women in birth in Africa, France, and the UK. She has worked as a lawyer and human rights lawyer for the last 18 years, and her work has brought her in touch with women and children. Kerry has spent the last 12 years living in the South of France and qualified as a Birth Doula and breastfeeding support assistant. Kerry served as vice-president of Allaitement Votre, a breastfeeding support group in France for two years. She has recently moved to Canada where she trained as a HypnoBirthing® Practitioner. Kerry teaches prenatal and babycare classes at Sunnybrook hospital. She is the mother of five and lives with her husband and children in Toronto.

Melissa Harley

Melissa has been working with birthing women since bearing witness to the vaginal birth of her twin nieces in early 2002. As a doula, Melissa has had the pleasure to support more than 100 women and their families during birth. She is a DONA International Doula Trainer, DONA International SPAR (Florida representative), and DONA International Certification Committee Member. Melissa works as a Lamaze Certified Childbirth Educator, empowering women to listen to their inner voice and acknowledge their own strength to birth. Melissa and her husband Ken live in Tallahassee, Florida and have two children. mharley@capitalcitydoulaservices.com, www.capitalcitydoulaservices.com

Keshia Kamphuis

Keshia is a naturopathic doctor and certified doula with DONA International. She graduated from the Canadian College of Naturopathic Medicine in Toronto, Ontario in 2012 and has plans to open a practice in Edmonton, Alberta in 2012. Keshia's passion for women's health and commitment to volunteer has inspired travel to rural Guatemala and northern Haiti to support indigenous women prenatally and in birth. Find Keshia at www.drkeshia.com.

Crescence Krueger

Crescence helps women in Toronto give birth, trains and mentors doulas and yoga teachers, and writes about it. Giving birth to her daughter at home in 1991 started it all. Her ability to integrate feminine wisdom into our current teaching and birthing environments is supported by the simple and profound yoga she has received from Mark Whitwell and the equally powerful connection to Isabel Perez and Isabel's teacher, Ina May Gaskin. Her writing has been published in *Bearing Witness: Childbirth Stories Told by Doulas*, edited by Lisa Doran and Lisa Caron, and in Mark Whitwell's *The Promise of Love, Sex and Intimacy*. www.heartofbirth.org

Jana Lok

Jana is a Registered Nurse with a passion for complementary therapies and holistic health practices. Having a highly experienced doula support her through two disparate birth experiences has shown her the importance of doula care in promoting best outcomes. She lives with her tech-savvy husband, two wonderful children, and one rambunctious but loyal Labrador retriever in Markham, Ontario.

Millennia (Millie) Lytle

Millennia Lytle ND, MPH, attended births from 2002 to 2012 as part of her naturopathic practice in Toronto, Ontario. Since finishing her Master's degree in Public Health in Germany, she has been concentrating on the integration of traditional, complementary, and alternative medicine (TCAM) into varying healthcare systems in Canada and internationally. Millie became a doula a year before she got her ND license. She just couldn't wait to see the babies. www.milliesays.com or www.facebook.com/Milliesays

Mona Mathews

Mona is a DONA certified birth doula. She came to this work after raising two daughters and working in the corporate world for 25 years. Working with families, empowering women to believe in themselves and their ability to give birth, has been her greatest accomplishment to date. What she did not realize when starting this journey is that their strength and stamina is reciprocal. Empowering women has empowered her! She is living a serendipitous life at a cottage on McRae Beach, Ontario with the love of her life of 38 years and their dog Rodney. www.newmarketdoula.ca

Nicole McKay

Nicole McKay is a birth and postpartum doula, childbirth educator, and La Leche League Leader. She supports growing families in Toronto with pregnancy, birth, and breastfeeding as they get in touch with the deep wisdom of their own mind, body, and spirit. She is honored and grateful to be invited to share in these journeys with so many families and looks forward to helping more women discover their inner birth goddess. Nicole and her husband Jamie are the proud parents of two children – Siobhan and Cayden. www.birthgoddess.ca

Hilary Monk

Hilary is the mother of four children, three born at home before the licensing of midwifery in Ontario. She is a former 'lay' and licensed midwife, Middle Eastern dancer, vajrayana Buddhist practitioner, perennial political pariah, and phronetic researcher. From her paradise base in Prince Edward County, Ontario, she completed a Master of Arts degree studying the lack of midwives freedom to follow client choices. Currently, she is studying at the Faculty of Business and Law at the University of the West of England. hilary.college@yahoo.ca.

Alicia Montgomery

Alicia is a birth doula, CD (DONA), and childbirth educator. Her birth work began in 2006 with a desire to help women feel as strong and powerful during their birth experiences as she did during her own. She attended Birthing From Within® Mentor Workshop in 2008 to expand her tools to help women through the emotional journey of birth. Now she hosts birthing classes year round. She lives with her four wonderfully wild sons (three born in hospital, one at home), her dedicated husband, and their cat in Novi, Michigan. www.cradleofbirth.com alicia@cradleofbirth.com

Beth Murch

Beth is a tree-hugging, crunchy-granola social justice activist who works as a full-spectrum doula and independent placenta service provider in Kitchener, Ontario. A spoken word artist who has competed nationally, she can be found creating and disturbing the peace through her literary craft which draws upon themes of sexuality, nature, spirituality, and feminism. Beth's life-long goal is to study midwifery and to become a wizened-old lady who lives at the edge of the woods, calling forth Buddhas from their mothers' wombs, healing with mysterious herbs, wearing feathers and bones in her dreadlocks, and reading palms and tea leaves. beth.murch@gmail.com

Christa Niravong

Christa is the mother of two young children, Atarah and Akadius. She is a graduate of McGill University, a La Leche League Leader, and founded an Elimination Communication Group in Guelph, Ontario. She has been featured in the news and in the documentary, *My Toxic Baby*. She is currently self-employed along with her husband Frederick in an adventure zipline company in Elora, Ontario.

Barbara Pal

The mother of three children, Barbara has been a birth and post-partum doula since 2008 in Toronto. She believes birth is a natural, healthy experience, not an illness or medical emergency. Barbara supports women in their birthing, feeding, and parenting choices, believing there is more than one right way to raise a child. Barbara likes to cook, hike, walk in the rain with her kids, laugh, and eat chocolate. www.dancingdoulatoronto.com or email dancing-doula@rogers.com.

Jennifer Papaconstantinou

Jennifer is a graduate of the Institute of Holistic Nutrition in Toronto, where she earned her designation as a Certified Holistic Nutritionist. She decided to pursue her passion as a health educator after successfully experiencing first-hand the profound effects of diet and lifestyle in creating balance and health within her own family. Jennifer realized the effects of diet on health while running a home daycare center for 15 years and witnessing directly the deterioration of the health of our next generation. Jennifer lives in Pickering, Ontario, with her husband Chris, who cherish raising their four beautiful children. www.healnaturally.ca www.growinghealthykids.ca

Kirsten Perley

Kirsten graduated from McMaster University in 1999 with a Bachelor of Science degree in Nursing and worked as a labor and delivery nurse at a Toronto hospital before leaving to study at a naturopathic college. For the past five years she has been co-teaching the Maternal Newborn Care Course at the Canadian College of Naturopathic Medicine. Body Works Center Newmarket ON www.bodyworkscenter.ca

Joanne Raines

Joanne's interest in birth began as an adolescent. Before the word "doula" was known to her, she accompanied her first birthing mom. Joanne's practice, Whispering Heart Doula Services, spans the York Region and Toronto. As a CAPPA Certified Childbirth Educator, DONA Certified Birth Doula, Postpartum Doula, member of many organizations, former Director then President of Doula-CARE, Joanne offers prenatal classes, guidance, and support to expectant and new families so they can welcome their babies with confidence.

Jenny Repec

Jenny lives in Toronto with her family. Although she knows how crucial it is to sleep when the baby sleeps, she felt compelled to tell her story and often wrote instead! Jenny has worked in a variety of fields, ranging from environmental activism to her own organic bakery, to fine art and antiques. Her own wonderful experience of pregnancy and the birth of her son has made her an advocate of birthing centers in Ontario, with the hope that all women will have the chance to choose a natural birth in an appropriate and peaceful setting.

Mary Sharpe

Mary Sharpe, RM BA MEd PhD, is a Registered Midwife, Associate Professor, and Director of the Ryerson Midwifery Education Program (MEP). In the early 1970s, Mary began working as a birth attendant, childbirth educator, and lactation consultant. She has been a practicing midwife in Ontario since 1979, and since 1994, has taught in the Ryerson MEP. Her research interests include: changes in midwives' practices following regulation (Sharpe MEd 1995); woman-midwife relationships (PhD 2004); GBS intrapartum prophylaxis; Ontario midwifery data; and midwife-led home births.

Mary has six children and has had the grand privilege of acting as midwife for six of her eight grandchildren.

Michelle Sliva

Michelle resides in Markham, Ontario with her husband and three fuzzy cats that enjoy staring at her son at a safe distance. When not playing with her beloved son, Michelle teaches at an elementary school as an instrumental music teacher. Michelle also enjoys sewing, baking, shopping, playing the piano, and chasing her cats. Her husband is a piano teacher, so there is a lot of music in her home. She hopes her birth story will encourage pregnant women to seek the support of a doula. Email: mamich100@hotmail.com

Kendra Smith

Kendra Smith, Naturopathic Doctor, Birth Doula (DONA), and Reiki Master, practices in Collingwood, Ontario. Kendra grew up in the countryside surrounded by animals and nature where her lifelong passion for natural healing began. After completing her Kinesiology degree, she spent a year working as a Reiki practitioner in the Mountains of British Columbia, snowboarding, and practicing yoga daily before returning home to become a naturopathic doctor. Kendra's general family practice has a special interest in maternal newborn care and pediatrics. kendrahealthyliving@gmail.com kendrahealthyliving.wix.com/ks

Carla Tonelli

Carla is a Toronto journalist and the mother of three children. She's also a wife, a daughter, a sister, a cyclist, and a lapsed vegetarian. She is a huge fan of midwives everywhere. Twitter at @carla_tonelli.

Sofie Weber

Sofie is a mother, a wife, a daughter, a sister, a friend and a doula in Orangeville, Ontario. I have had the honor of watching birth unfold and I am blessed to have been able to take this journey.

Cady Williams

Cady is a home birth and postpartum doula and photographer. A life-long advocate for women's health and reproductive rights, she also co-founded an outdoor daycare center, was actively involved in a cooperative school, and lived and raised children in a collective household. Cady was, for many years, an organizer in the struggle for an independent Canada, financing her activism with a handful of interesting occupations. She is happy to be working with families and babies again. She lives in Toronto. cadywilliams-doula@gmail.com

Nicola Wolters

Having been a doula for 10 years and a mother for longer, Nicola is fascinated with the evolving identity of women as they transition from young woman to wife/partner to young mother, experienced mother and beyond, and how this changing identity impacts their careers, relationships, and beliefs. She has studied wellness coaching and hypnosis to compliment these interests.

Acknowledgments

As our call for authors traveled the world, we were so humbled and grateful each time we received a story. Especially as each story seemed to flow naturally into one another creating the perfect beginning, middle and end of this book, as if we had worked together planning it out. Our contributors are a group of wonderful women – mothers, doulas, and midwives, who shared their stories generously to give us a glimpse into the most intimate and powerful parts of their lives. Our contributing authors are, each in their own way, leaders and teachers in our field and share valuable narrative experiences that we can all learn from. Thank you so very much to all of you for your hard work and contributions to this book.

There are always elders in the field who inspire and encourage us. We wish to thank Penny Simkin, the mother of the doula movement, for her encouragement and ongoing support with the work of writing our books. We also thank Penny for the pleasure of her company as she shared her wisdom and experience at an intimate workshop in Toronto in 2012. We wish toe recognize with gratitude Ina May Gaskin for the weekend she spent sharing her ideas and philosophies so generously with the Toronto birth community in 2011. Stories inspired by Ina May that weekend pepper this book. We wish to extend a very special thank you to Mary Sharpe for her feedback, her experience, her clarity, and her willingness to participate in this project by authoring the foreword to this book. We are blessed to have such wise and experienced women in our lives that are willing to engage intensely in our ideas and vision.

We both wish to thank all of the incredible authors, thinkers, teachers, and world experts in the field of birth who read this book, generously gifted their time and their names and words of praise. Penny Simkin, Michel Odent, and Ann Douglas – thank you all so very much.

Our thanks go out as well to our publisher Bob Hilderley at Fox Women's Books for his enthusiasm for this project and for recognizing the value of women's stories of birth in their own voices.

Lisa Caron would like to thank ... my "book doulas" – Debbie Acacio, Lindsay Benjamin, Nuala Byles, Leslie Chandler, Jessica Cherniak, Jennifer Elliott, Tena McKenzie, Daniel Monroy Hernandez, Catherine Tammaro, and Macy Wilcken for their patience, support, and guidance during my precipitous book labors. And especially Lisa Doran for her inspirational clarity and endless patience.

Lisa Doran would like to thank...the Doran boys and their dad for their support of this project, especially when mom needed to disappear into the wilds for a few days to pull it all together, Mary King for the use of her dock on Potters Creek because the idea for this book was midwifed there, and Lisa Caron for willingly being part of the Lisa & Lisa dynamic duo, for her unending patience, sometimes unbelievable calm, and insistence that deadlines are important.